NEONATAL-PERINATAL BOARD REVIEW QUESTION BANK

Volume 5 of 5

Preparation Strategy, Mock Examinations, and Reference Appendix

Time Management, Self-Assessment, Psychological Readiness, and Practice Testing

First Edition, 2026

Author

Dr. Ahmed Badawy

MRCPCH (UK) | EBP | EPIC Diploma

ORCID 0009-0007-7662-840X

"Mechanism first. Honest about uncertainty. Connected across every chapter and every volume."

Talented LLC | Sheridan, Wyoming, USA

Copyright and Disclaimer

This question bank is intended as an educational review resource for physicians and trainees preparing for postgraduate neonatal-perinatal medicine certifying examinations. It is not a substitute for clinical judgement, institutional protocol, or direct patient assessment, and it does not constitute medical advice. The content reflects a synthesis of major guidelines and peer-reviewed literature current as of early 2026. Medicine changes continually; readers must consult the current version of the relevant guideline and current product information before making any treatment decision.

The author and publisher disclaim liability for any adverse consequence arising from the use or application of the information contained in this volume.

First Edition: 2026. Published by Talented LLC, Sheridan, Wyoming, USA.

Library of Congress Control Number (LCCN): 2026923203.

ISBN: 979-8-952203-09-9.

For permission requests: a.m.b.hassane@gmail.com

Printed in the United States of America.

Acknowledgements

This question bank was built across five volumes and many months, and it owes a debt to every clinician, researcher, and guideline body whose published, current work it draws upon and cites throughout. I am grateful to the neonatal-perinatal community whose ongoing, rigorous research makes a resource like this possible at all, and to the trainees and colleagues whose questions, in the truest sense, shaped every question in this book.

To my family, whose patience made the space for this work: thank you.

How to Use This Volume

Volume 5 closes this series with the material that surrounds the clinical content itself: how to manage your study time, how to measure your own genuine readiness, how to steady yourself psychologically through exam week, three complete and fully independent mock examinations, a list of valuable further reading, and a reference ranges appendix for quick, ongoing use.

Read the three preparation-strategy chapters early in your overall study period, not only in the final week — the guidance on spaced repetition, blueprint tracking, and mock-exam pacing is considerably more useful when there is still time left to act on it.

The three mock examinations are entirely independent of one another and of every chapter in Volumes 1 through 4 — no vignette or correct answer repeats. Take them spaced apart, under real timed conditions, and use the guidance in this volume's own second chapter to interpret your results diagnostically rather than as a single pass-or-fail verdict.

The reference ranges appendix is built to be used, not read once — keep it close during the remainder of your preparation and at the bedside afterward.

Table of Contents

Chapter: Time Management Strategies to Succeed

There are two entirely different time-management problems hiding inside exam preparation, and most candidates only ever plan for one of them. The first is the slow, months-long problem: how do you allocate a genuinely limited number of study hours across seventeen chapters and three volumes of material without either running out of time or burning out halfway through. The second is the fast, minutes-long problem: how do you move through 200-plus questions in a fixed number of hours without a single, difficult question quietly costing you the ten easy questions that came after it. This chapter treats both, in that order.

1. Building the Study Schedule

Work backward from the exam date, not forward from today. Count the weeks you genuinely have, subtract a final week reserved for light review only, and divide what remains across this book's own blueprint weighting rather than evenly across chapters. A chapter with 210 questions represents roughly five times the content weight of a chapter with 45 questions, and your study hours should roughly track that same proportion, not an equal number of days per chapter regardless of size.

Active recall beats re-reading, and this is not a close contest. Reading a chapter a second or third time creates a genuine, but misleading, sense of familiarity — recognising a fact when you see it again is a considerably easier cognitive task than producing that same fact from memory when a vignette demands it, and the exam only ever asks for the second, harder task. Treat every chapter's own closing synthesis questions and every subdomain's blueprint tracker as your primary study tool, not as an afterthought completed once at the end. Work a chapter once for understanding, then return to its questions repeatedly, spaced across subsequent weeks, rather than moving on and never returning.

A Practical Weekly Structure

Four to five substantive study sessions per week, each 90 to 150 minutes, is genuinely more effective than daily, shorter sessions that never reach deep engagement with a single topic.

Reserve one full day most weeks with no formal study at all. This is not lost time — consolidation of learned material happens substantially during rest and sleep, and a schedule with no recovery built in reliably degrades in its final weeks, precisely when performance matters most.

Revisit, don't just advance. Roughly one session in four should return to material covered two or more weeks earlier, rather than moving continuously forward through new content. Spaced repetition is not a nice-to-have technique; it is the single best-evidenced method for converting short-term recognition into long-term, retrievable knowledge.

2. A Sample Countdown Timeline

This is a template, not a prescription — adjust the specific weeks to your own, actual calendar and starting point. The proportions matter more than the exact week numbers.

Weeks 1 through 60% of your total preparation window: work through Volumes 1 through 3 chapter by chapter, in order, completing every question in each chapter and its closing synthesis before advancing. Do not skip a chapter's harder subdomain because it feels slower — slower usually means it is where you are genuinely learning something new, which is precisely where your time should go.

Next 20% of your window: take Mock Examination 1 under real timed conditions. Score it honestly by section, identify your two or three weakest subdomains specifically (not just "I did badly"), and spend the following days returning to those specific chapters rather than restudying everything indiscriminately.

Next 15% of your window: take Mock Examination 2. Compare your section-by-section performance directly against Mock Examination 1. A persistent weak section across both exams is your single clearest, most reliable signal of where remaining time belongs. A section that improved meaningfully tells you your targeted restudy worked — keep doing more of it elsewhere.

Final stretch, roughly the last 5% of your window: take Mock Examination 3, then stop introducing new material entirely. Use the remaining days for light, targeted review of your own weakest points only, adequate sleep, and the exam-week strategy in a later chapter of this volume. Cramming unfamiliar material in the final 48 hours reliably produces worse outcomes than consolidating what you already, genuinely know.

3. Pacing During the Actual Examination

Calculate your own, specific per-question time budget before you sit down, and know it cold. If your examination allots, for example, four hours to 200 questions, that is 72 seconds per question on average — but averages hide the real skill. The genuine skill is recognising, within the first 20 to 30 seconds of reading a question, whether you know it, are unsure but can reason your way there, or are genuinely stuck, and then acting differently in each of those three cases.

The Three-Bucket Rule

If you know it: answer and move on. Do not re-read a question you already, confidently answered — this is one of the most common sources of wasted time and, worse, of a correct answer changed to a wrong one under second-guessing pressure.

If you can reason your way there: work it, using the process-of-elimination habits this book's own "wrong answer" explanations have modelled throughout — identify the specific reason each wrong option fails, rather than searching for the right answer in isolation. Give yourself a firm cap, roughly double your average per-question time, then commit to your best answer and move on.

If you are genuinely stuck: flag it, select your best guess as a placeholder rather than leaving it blank, and move on immediately. A blank answer is guaranteed wrong; a guess has genuine odds. Never let one unfamiliar question consume the time budget of the next five familiar ones.

Build in checkpoints. If you have four hours for 200 questions, you should be at question 50 by the one-hour mark, question 100 by two hours, and so on. Check your position against the clock at each checkpoint, not only at the very end — by the time you discover you are 40 questions behind schedule with 20 minutes left, there is very little left to do about it.

Reserve your final 10 to 15 minutes exclusively for flagged questions, not for re-reading answers you already feel settled about. Revisit only what you genuinely marked as uncertain, and resist the urge to open a new, difficult question you have not yet seen with almost no time left to actually work it properly.

Chapter: Measuring Your Own Readiness

How to Know When You're Actually Ready, Not Just Tired of Studying

1. Why Self-Assessment Is Genuinely Hard

Most candidates do not overestimate or underestimate their own readiness because they are careless. They do it because the brain's own sense of familiarity is a poor, and frequently misleading, proxy for actual, retrievable knowledge. Re-reading a chapter you have already studied produces a genuine, felt sense of "yes, I know this" — recognising a fact is easy. But an examination never asks you to recognise a fact sitting in front of you; it asks you to produce the correct reasoning from memory, under time pressure, embedded in a vignette designed to look like several other, similar conditions. That gap, between recognition and recall, is exactly where a comfortable feeling of readiness and an actual, safe level of readiness quietly diverge.

The reverse distortion is just as real. A single difficult mock exam, or a stretch of several genuinely hard questions in a row, can produce a wave of underconfidence entirely disproportionate to what it actually reflects about your overall preparation. Both errors point to the same underlying fix: replace how you feel about your own readiness with a small number of concrete, structured signals you can actually track over time.

2. Reading Your Own Blueprint Score Trackers Correctly

Every chapter in this book's own question bank ends with a blueprint score tracker organised by subdomain, not as a single, aggregate percentage. This structure exists for a specific, deliberate reason: a single overall score of 75 per cent can hide a genuinely dangerous pattern — 95 per cent in four subdomains and 40 per cent in a fifth — just as easily as it can reflect a genuinely even, moderate grasp across the board. Only the subdomain breakdown tells you which of these two, very different situations you are actually in.

How to Use a Subdomain Tracker Honestly

Record your score by subdomain every time, not just your total. A single number discards the most useful information the tracker was built to give you.

Distinguish a persistent gap from a one-off miss. Getting two questions wrong in a subdomain you otherwise handled well is normal variation. Getting most questions wrong in the same subdomain across two or more separate chapters, or across a chapter and a later mock exam, is a genuine, structural gap that deserves focused, deliberate return — not just "try harder next time."

Re-test the same subdomain after targeted review, rather than assuming a single round of rereading fixed it. If you missed several acid-base questions, restudy that specific content, then deliberately seek out further acid-base questions — across other chapters that connect to it — to confirm the gap actually closed, rather than simply feeling more familiar with the material.

3. Using the Three Mock Examinations Diagnostically

This book's three mock examinations were deliberately built as independent, non-overlapping instruments — no vignette or correct answer repeats across them — specifically so that your performance across all three, taken together, tells you something a single exam cannot. A single mock exam score is one data point; three scores, tracked across sections, is a trend.

Look for a stable core score band rather than a single peak. If your overall score across all three mock exams sits within a narrow band — say, within five or six percentage points of each other — that consistency is itself meaningful information: it suggests your actual, retrievable knowledge has stabilised, rather than one strong result being a lucky draw of questions you happened to know well. A single excellent score surrounded by two considerably weaker ones is a less reliable signal of true readiness than three consistent, moderate scores.

Track section-level trends across all three exams side by side — Foundations, Organ Systems, and Application — not just the overall total. A section that improves meaningfully from Mock 1 to Mock 3 tells you that targeted restudy is working and should continue. A section that stays weak across all three exams despite genuine, targeted effort is the single clearest, most trustworthy signal in this entire book of exactly where your remaining preparation time belongs.

Take at least one mock examination under genuinely realistic conditions: a single sitting, timed, without pausing to look anything up. Practising the actual, physical and mental experience of sustained exam-length concentration is itself a skill this book's own content cannot teach through untimed, chapter-by-chapter review alone.

4. A Concrete Readiness Checklist

No single checklist can substitute for genuine judgement about your own, individual preparation, but the following signals, taken together, distinguish a candidate who is genuinely ready from one who needs more time considerably more reliably than a felt sense of confidence alone.

Signs You Are Likely Genuinely Ready

Your subdomain scores across every chapter's blueprint tracker are consistently at or above your own, personal target threshold, with no subdomain persistently and significantly below the others.

Your overall score across all three mock examinations sits in a stable, narrow band, rather than one high outlier surrounded by two considerably weaker results.

When you get a mock-exam question wrong, you can usually identify, on review, the specific, precise reasoning gap that caused it — rather than the error feeling arbitrary or unexplainable.

You can complete a full, timed mock examination within the allotted time with a genuine reserve of a few minutes for a final review pass, rather than rushing the final quarter of the exam.

Signs You Likely Need More Time

One or more specific subdomains remain persistently weak across multiple, separate chapters or exams despite genuine, targeted review — not just a single, isolated miss.

Your mock examination scores are trending downward, rather than stable or improving, across your later attempts.

You consistently run out of time before completing a full, timed mock examination, rather than finishing with time to spare.

Reviewing a wrong answer regularly leaves you unable to explain why the correct answer was correct, even after reading the explanation — this suggests a genuine, underlying gap in mechanism-level understanding, not simply an unlucky question.

5. What a Single Bad Mock Exam Does and Doesn't Mean

A single, disappointing mock examination result is data, not a verdict. Test performance genuinely varies session to session for reasons that have nothing to do with your actual, underlying knowledge — sleep the night before, an unusually clustered run of your own weaker subdomains appearing more often than they statistically should in that particular 60-question sample, or simple, ordinary variance. One weak result does not undo months of consistent, structured preparation, and it should not be treated as though it does.

What a single weak result should genuinely prompt is exactly the structured review this chapter has described throughout: look at the section breakdown, not just the total; identify whether the weakness is genuinely new or a known, persistent pattern reasserting itself; and use it to direct your remaining study time rather than to catastrophise about your overall preparation. The candidates who use a disappointing mock exam as a specific, targeted diagnostic tool tend to walk into the real examination considerably better prepared than candidates who either ignore a weak result or let it derail their confidence entirely.

Chapter: Steadying Yourself

Psychological Preparation and Exam-Week Strategy

A note before this chapter begins: what follows is general, evidence-informed guidance on managing ordinary exam-related stress — the kind nearly every candidate for a genuinely demanding certifying examination experiences. It is not a substitute for professional mental health care. If you are dealing with anxiety, low mood, or stress that feels significant, persistent, or bigger than the exam itself, reaching out to a therapist, counsellor, or your own physician is a genuinely valuable, appropriate step — not a sign that you are somehow less prepared or less capable than anyone else sitting this examination.

1. Reframing What Exam-Day Nerves Actually Are

The physical sensations of exam anxiety — a racing heart, a tight chest, restless energy — are, physiologically, nearly identical to the sensations of excitement and readiness. The body cannot easily tell the difference between "I am threatened" and "something important is about to happen and I am mobilised for it"; the interpretation is supplied by the mind, not the body. A body of research on stress reappraisal has found that people who are coached to consciously relabel these same physical sensations — "my body is preparing me to perform," rather than "I am panicking" — often go on to perform measurably better under pressure than those who try to suppress or fight the sensation entirely.

This is worth genuinely internalising before exam week arrives, not discovering for the first time in the exam hall: a racing pulse before a big exam is not evidence that something is wrong. It is closer to evidence that you understand exactly how much this moment matters. The goal is not to eliminate the feeling; it is to stop treating the feeling itself as a problem.

2. The Final Week: Tapering, Not Cramming

The single most consistent finding across performance psychology, in academic testing and in athletics alike, is that a taper — a deliberate reduction in workload in the final days before a peak performance — produces better outcomes than pushing volume all the way to the finish line. Muscles and minds alike consolidate what they have already built during rest, not during additional strain piled on top of an already-full tank.

A Practical Final-Week Structure

Six to seven days out: your last full day of substantive new-material study. After this point, shift entirely to review of material you have already covered — no new chapters, no new subdomains.

Three to four days out: review only your own, specific weak points identified from your blueprint trackers and mock exam section scores. Resist the pull to re-read entire chapters end to end; targeted review of known gaps is a considerably better use of these final days.

Two days out: light review only, no more than an hour or two, followed by something genuinely unrelated to studying — exercise, time with people you care about, anything that lets your mind rest.

The day before: no studying at all, if you can manage it. Confirm logistics — exam location, required documents, what time you need to leave — early in the day so none of it is left for the anxious hours before bed. Prioritise sleep over one final review pass; a well-rested mind consistently outperforms a slightly-more-reviewed but exhausted one.

3. Sleep Is Not Optional

Of every single piece of exam-week advice in this chapter, this is the one with the strongest, most consistent evidence behind it: sleep loss measurably degrades working memory, sustained attention, and exactly the kind of multi-step clinical reasoning this examination is built to test. Sacrificing sleep for one additional night of review is, for the overwhelming majority of candidates, a losing trade — you are not gaining more than you are giving up. Protect seven to eight hours nightly for at least the final week, and treat this as seriously as any other part of your preparation, not as a luxury to sacrifice when time feels short.

4. Practical Techniques for the Acute Moment

Some tools are for the days beforehand; others are for the specific, acute moment — the minute before the exam starts, or the moment mid-exam when a difficult question spikes your anxiety and threatens to carry into the next five questions with it.

Before the Exam Begins

Slow, extended exhale breathing. A pattern such as inhaling for four counts and exhaling for six to eight is one of the most reliably, quickly effective ways to lower acute physiological arousal, since a longer exhale relative to inhale directly activates the body's own calming response. A few minutes of this before you sit down is genuinely worth the time.

Arrive with margin. Rushing in at the last possible minute adds an entirely avoidable layer of stress on top of the exam itself. Build in more transit and check-in time than you think you need.

Have a brief, specific mental script ready — a sentence or two you say to yourself, silently, right before starting. Something concrete and true, such as "I have prepared for this specific exam for months; I know how to work through a question I don't immediately recognise." A vague hope ("I'll be fine") is considerably less effective than a specific, evidence-based reminder of your own actual preparation.

If You Blank or Spiral Mid-Exam

Name it, then move. Silently acknowledging "I'm anxious right now" takes far less time than fighting the feeling, and tends to loosen its grip faster than trying to suppress it.

Use the three-bucket rule from the preceding chapter on time management: if a specific question has you stuck, flag it, select your best guess, and move to the next question immediately. Physically moving forward interrupts the spiral considerably more effectively than staring at the same, stuck question.

Take three slow breaths, extended exhale, before starting the very next question. This costs perhaps fifteen seconds and reliably prevents one difficult question from degrading your performance on the several questions that follow it.

Remember that a difficult run of two or three questions in a row is expected, ordinary exam experience, not a sign the exam is somehow "going badly." Every candidate sitting this examination hits a stretch like this at some point; it is not diagnostic of your overall performance.

5. The Morning of the Examination

Eat something, even if you do not feel hungry — stable blood glucose supports sustained concentration over several hours considerably better than an empty stomach does. Avoid a substantially different caffeine dose than your normal routine, in either direction; both a large, unfamiliar increase and an abrupt withdrawal can meaningfully affect focus and anxiety on exactly the day you need neither.

Do a light, brief review at most — skimming your own summary notes or a single blueprint tracker, not opening a new chapter. The goal of the morning is confidence reinforcement, not last-minute learning; genuinely new material absorbed in the final hour before an exam is rarely retained and frequently adds anxiety rather than reducing it.

Finally: you have, by this point, worked through this entire book's own five volumes, its blueprint trackers, and three complete mock examinations. That is a genuinely substantial, structured body of preparation, not a hope. Walk in trusting the work you have already, actually done.

Mock Examination 1

A Comprehensive, Cross-Volume Practice Examination

60 Questions — Foundations, Organ Systems, and Application Together

A Different Kind of Chapter

Every chapter in this book so far has taught. This exam tests. The questions that follow are entirely new — not drawn from any earlier chapter — and they are written in the genuine, clinical-vignette format the actual certifying examination itself uses: a patient presentation, relevant findings, and a single best answer, rather than the "which statement is most accurate" format this book has used throughout its own teaching content.

This exam is proportionally weighted to reflect this entire book's own five-volume structure: a foundations section drawing on Volume 1's physiological and pharmacological groundwork, a substantial organ systems section drawing on Volumes 2 and 3's comprehensive, system-by-system content, and an application section drawing on Volume 4's surgical, transport, systems, ethical, and biostatistical content. Many questions deliberately require synthesis across more than one volume at once — exactly as the real examination, and real clinical practice, actually demand.

How to Use This Exam

Work through all 60 questions in a single, timed sitting if possible — the actual certifying examination rewards stamina as well as knowledge. A reasonable target is roughly 90 seconds per question, or about 90 minutes total.

Resist the urge to check the answer after each question. This exam is formatted with the explanation immediately following each question for ease of review afterward, but genuine practice value comes from committing to an answer before reading further.

Score yourself by section, not only as a single total. A weak foundations section points to different revision than a weak application section.

A Note on Figures

Every figure in this book is original artwork, drawn specifically for it. No stock images, no licensed photographs and no third-party illustrations are used anywhere in the text.

Questions

Section A: Foundations (Questions 1-9) — Section B: Organ Systems (Questions 10–50) — Section C: Application (Questions 51–60)

Question 1

A 24-year-old primigravida at 23 weeks 4 days gestation presents with painless cervical dilation and is found to have a cervical length of 8 mm on transvaginal ultrasound, with visible membrane bulging. She and her partner meet with the neonatology and maternal-fetal medicine teams together to discuss the range of options available should preterm birth become imminent within the next several days. Which of the following best describes the correct approach to this specific counselling conversation?

A. The neonatology team should independently determine and recommend a single, preferred management plan, then present this plan to the family as the only medically appropriate option

B. The family should be presented with the complete, honest range of options, including comfort-focused care, active resuscitation, and the genuine uncertainty in outcome prediction at this specific gestational age, through a coordinated, shared decision-making conversation involving both obstetric and neonatal teams together

C. Because 23 weeks 4 days falls below the threshold of viability in every circumstance, only comfort-focused care should be offered

D. The family's own values and preferences are not relevant to this specific decision, which should be made entirely on the basis of gestational age alone

E. This conversation should be deferred entirely until after delivery, since antenatal counselling provides no genuine benefit at this specific gestational age

Answer: B. **This is a periviability counselling scenario requiring coordinated, honest, shared decision-making — presenting the complete range of options with genuine uncertainty acknowledged, rather than a single, unilaterally determined recommendation.**

At 23 weeks 4 days, this pregnancy sits within the genuinely uncertain periviable window in which outcome prediction carries considerable, honest uncertainty and where professional guidance consistently supports shared, rather than unilateral, decision-making.

The correct approach directly integrates this book's own repeated, foundational principles: coordinated obstetric-neonatal counselling, honest acknowledgement of genuine prognostic uncertainty at this specific gestational age, and presentation of the complete range of reasonable options — comfort-focused care and active resuscitation alike — rather than a single, clinician-determined path.

This reflects the same shared decision-making framework established throughout this book's own ethics content: parents deserve complete, honest information and genuine partnership in this decision, not a predetermined recommendation presented as the only acceptable choice.

Why the other options are wrong

A. Unilateral determination contradicts the shared decision-making principle this entire scenario requires.

C. This specific gestational age falls within a genuinely uncertain, not uniformly non-viable, window requiring individualised discussion.

D. A family's own values and preferences are genuinely central to this specific decision, not irrelevant.

E. Antenatal counselling provides genuine, substantial value precisely because it occurs before delivery, allowing structured planning.

Board Alert Periviability counselling at 22–24 weeks requires coordinated, shared decision-making with honest acknowledgement of genuine outcome uncertainty — never a single, unilaterally presented recommendation.

Mock Exam 1 — Section A: Foundations | Universal Task 4: Management, Treatment and Prevention

Question 2

A term infant is delivered via spontaneous vaginal delivery and at 30 seconds of life is noted to have poor respiratory effort, a heart rate of 90 beats per minute by auscultation, and diffuse cyanosis. The umbilical cord has not yet been clamped. Which of the following represents the most appropriate next step, according to the current Neonatal Resuscitation Program algorithm?

A. Immediately clamp and cut the umbilical cord, then proceed directly to chest compressions

B. Begin positive pressure ventilation while deferring cord clamping if the equipment and personnel required to do so safely are genuinely available

C. Administer intravenous epinephrine immediately, prior to any attempt at establishing effective ventilation

D. Provide only free-flow oxygen and reassess in five minutes without further intervention

E. Immediately intubate this infant prior to any attempt at mask ventilation, regardless of this infant's own response to initial, less invasive support

Answer: B. **This infant demonstrates inadequate respiratory effort and a heart rate below 100, meeting criteria for positive pressure ventilation as the immediate next step — with cord management now positioned as this algorithm's own first consideration where equipment and personnel genuinely allow deferred clamping alongside initial support.**

The current Neonatal Resuscitation Program algorithm establishes ventilation, not chest compressions or medication, as the single most important, effective intervention in neonatal resuscitation, and this infant's heart rate of 90 with poor respiratory effort meets the specific threshold for positive pressure ventilation.

Cord management now sits as this algorithm's own initial consideration: where the necessary equipment and personnel are genuinely available, deferred cord clamping alongside initial respiratory support represents current, evidence-based practice, rather than reflexively clamping and cutting before any resuscitative step.

Chest compressions are reserved for a heart rate below 60 despite effective ventilation for 30 seconds; epinephrine is reserved for continued bradycardia despite effective ventilation and compressions together — neither is indicated as an immediate, first step in this specific scenario.

Why the other options are wrong

A. Chest compressions are not indicated at this heart rate; ventilation is the correct, immediate priority.

C. Epinephrine is reserved for persistent bradycardia despite effective ventilation and compressions, not as an initial step.

D. This heart rate and respiratory effort meet criteria for positive pressure ventilation, not free-flow oxygen alone.

E. Mask ventilation is the appropriate initial approach; immediate intubation is not indicated before assessing response to less invasive support.

Board Alert Ventilation is the single most effective intervention in neonatal resuscitation. Current NRP guidance positions cord management as an initial consideration, supporting deferred clamping alongside initial support where feasible.

Question 3

A 29-week gestation infant is delivered and immediately placed in a polyethylene bag without drying, with a radiant warmer set to servo-control mode and a chemical warming mattress beneath. Despite these measures, the admission temperature is 35.2°C. Which of the following most directly explains the specific rationale for this combined, multimodal thermal approach, and what does this specific finding most appropriately prompt?

A. This combined approach targets a single mechanism of heat loss alone, and this finding reflects a normal, expected outcome requiring no further action

B. This combined approach targets multiple, distinct mechanisms of heat loss simultaneously — evaporation, convection, and conduction together — and this finding, despite these combined measures, should prompt active review of specific technique and environmental factors rather than assumption that further, additional intervention would be genuinely futile

C. Polyethylene wrapping alone eliminates all heat loss, making the additional warming mattress entirely unnecessary and redundant

D. This specific temperature is well within the accepted, normal range and reflects successful thermal management requiring no further consideration

E. Extremely preterm infants are expected to remain hypothermic despite optimal management, and this finding should not prompt any further, active review

Answer: B. This combined approach directly targets multiple, distinct mechanisms of heat loss simultaneously, and a genuinely elevated risk of hypothermia despite these measures should prompt active review of technique, not passive acceptance.

This multimodal approach directly reflects this book's own established thermal physiology: polyethylene wrapping without drying addresses evaporative loss, a warmed environment addresses convective loss, and a warming mattress addresses conductive loss — three genuinely distinct mechanisms requiring three genuinely distinct interventions.

An admission temperature of 35.2°C, despite this combined approach, falls below the target range and should actively prompt review of specific technique — was the bag genuinely sealed, was the warmer genuinely functioning, was transport time genuinely minimised — rather than assuming this outcome was genuinely unavoidable.

This population's own genuinely elevated surface-area-to-body-mass ratio and reduced subcutaneous insulation make thermal vulnerability genuinely significant, but this vulnerability is a reason for active, structured intervention and honest review when targets are missed, not passive acceptance of a suboptimal outcome.

Why the other options are wrong

A. This combined approach targets multiple, distinct mechanisms, not a single mechanism alone; this outcome warrants active review.

C. These three interventions address genuinely distinct mechanisms; none alone is sufficient to eliminate all heat loss.

D. This temperature falls below the accepted target range and does not reflect successful thermal management.

E. Active, structured intervention meaningfully reduces hypothermia risk in this population; this outcome should prompt review, not acceptance.

Board Alert Combined thermal interventions target genuinely distinct mechanisms of heat loss. A missed thermal target despite these measures should prompt active technique review, not passive acceptance.

Question 4

A 26-week gestation infant on day 3 of life is noted to have a blood pressure that is stable and appropriate for gestational age, with normal urine output and lactate. An echocardiogram performed for a separate indication incidentally demonstrates a left ventricle that appears to function normally despite reduced myofibrillar content relative to a term infant. Which of the following best explains why this infant's cardiac output remains adequate despite this specific, structural immaturity?

A. This infant's myocardium has already achieved full structural and functional maturity by day 3 of life, making this described finding inaccurate

B. This infant compensates through an increased reliance on heart rate, given a comparatively limited Frank-Starling reserve, while remaining more vulnerable to increased afterload than a term infant would be

C. This infant's cardiac output is entirely independent of heart rate, preload, and afterload alike at this specific gestational age

D. Reduced myofibrillar content has no genuine functional consequence of any kind in the preterm myocardium

E. This infant's myocardium is structurally identical to a term infant's myocardium, with no genuine developmental distinction between them

Answer: B. **The immature myocardium's own reduced myofibrillar content directly explains its genuinely limited Frank-Starling reserve and heart-rate-dependent compensation, while also explaining its genuinely elevated vulnerability to increased afterload.**

This vignette directly tests the three-part myocardial immaturity framework established throughout this book: reduced myofibrillar content structurally explains a genuinely limited preload response (Frank-Starling mechanism), a genuinely important reliance on heart rate (force-frequency relationship), and a genuinely elevated sensitivity to increased afterload (stress-velocity relationship).

This infant's adequate cardiac output despite structural immaturity directly reflects genuine, active compensation through this same, heart-rate-dependent mechanism, rather than reflecting that this infant's myocardium has somehow already achieved full, term-equivalent maturity.

This framework carries direct, practical bedside relevance: correctly understanding this same, structural immaturity explains why fluid boluses alone often provide limited benefit in this population, and why careful attention to systemic vascular resistance carries particular importance.

Why the other options are wrong

A. This infant's myocardium remains genuinely immature at this gestational age and postnatal day; this statement is inaccurate.

C. Cardiac output remains genuinely dependent on all three of these parameters, though the relative contribution of each differs from a term infant.

D. Reduced myofibrillar content carries genuine, specific functional consequence, as detailed in the correct answer.

E. A genuine, significant structural distinction exists between the preterm and term myocardium at this gestational age.

Board Alert Reduced myofibrillar content in the immature myocardium explains limited preload reserve, heart-rate-dependent compensation, and elevated afterload sensitivity together — a three-part framework with direct bedside relevance.

Question 5

A 31-week gestation infant on postnatal day 9 of mechanical ventilation has a blood gas showing pH 7.23, PCO2 65 mmHg, and a normal bicarbonate for gestational age. The clinical team is debating whether to escalate ventilator settings. Which of the following best reflects the current, evidence-based approach to this specific finding?

A. This blood gas reflects a primary metabolic disturbance requiring immediate correction with sodium bicarbonate

B. This blood gas reflects a primary respiratory disturbance that falls within a pH-controlled permissive hypercapnia range shown in current trial evidence to increase ventilator-free days without significant differences in bronchopulmonary dysplasia or neurodevelopmental harm, supporting continued, careful monitoring rather than reflexive escalation

C. Any PCO2 above 45 mmHg in a preterm infant mandates immediate ventilator escalation regardless of pH or clinical context

D. This finding has no established relationship to any current evidence regarding ventilator management strategy

E. The normal bicarbonate concentration indicates this infant requires no further monitoring of any kind

Answer: B. This blood gas — elevated PCO2 with normal bicarbonate — reflects a primary respiratory disturbance falling within a genuinely current, evidence-supported permissive hypercapnia target range associated with increased ventilator-free

days without significant harm.

The elevated PCO2 with normal bicarbonate for gestational age reflects a primary respiratory, rather than metabolic, disturbance — the classification principle underlying correct interpretation of any neonatal blood gas.

This specific pH and PCO2 combination falls within the higher, pH-controlled permissive hypercapnia target range established by a genuinely current randomised trial, which found this range associated with increased ventilator-free days during the 28 days following randomisation, without significant differences in bronchopulmonary dysplasia or evidence of neurodevelopmental harm on follow-up.

The genuinely current, honestly acknowledged absence of a formally established upper carbon dioxide safety limit supports continued, careful monitoring in this specific circumstance, rather than either uncritical reassurance or reflexive ventilator escalation.

Why the other options are wrong

A. This finding reflects a primary respiratory, not metabolic, disturbance; bicarbonate administration is not indicated here.

C. This specific PCO2 and pH combination falls within an evidence-supported target range; a rigid, universal threshold is not the correct approach.

D. This finding has direct, specific relevance to genuinely current permissive hypercapnia trial evidence, as detailed in the correct answer.

E. Continued, careful monitoring remains appropriate; a normal bicarbonate does not eliminate the need for ongoing attention.

Board Alert A genuinely current randomised trial found a higher, pH-controlled permissive hypercapnia target (pH ≥7.20, PCO2 60–75) associated with increased ventilator-free days, without significant BPD difference or neurodevelopmental harm.

Mock Exam 1 — Section A: Foundations | Universal Task 4: Management, Treatment and Prevention

Question 6

A 24-week gestation infant is receiving caffeine citrate for apnoea of prematurity and subsequently develops acute kidney injury. The clinical team is reconsidering the current caffeine dosing regimen. Which of the following best reflects current understanding of this clinical scenario?

A. Caffeine citrate has no established relationship to acute kidney injury of any kind, and this infant's renal status is entirely unrelated to this medication

B. Genuinely current research has identified an association between early caffeine citrate administration and acute kidney injury risk in preterm infants, and separately, genuinely current pharmacokinetic modelling has shown that the same, uniform weight-based dosing currently applied to every neonate does not account for differing renal function or gestational-age-specific metabolism, supporting individualised dosing consideration in this specific circumstance

C. Caffeine citrate should be immediately, permanently discontinued in every infant who develops acute kidney injury for any reason, regardless of ongoing apnoea of prematurity

D. This medication's dosing has already been fully individualised by gestational age and renal function in universal, current clinical practice

E. This infant's acute kidney injury provides no genuine information relevant to this medication's own future dosing

Answer: B. **Genuinely current research has identified a caffeine-AKI association, and separate, current pharmacokinetic modelling shows uniform dosing does not account for gestational-age-specific metabolism or renal function — supporting individualised dosing consideration here.**

This scenario directly reflects two, genuinely current, connected findings established throughout this book's pharmacology content: a genuinely current safety signal linking early caffeine citrate administration to acute kidney injury risk, and separate, current pharmacokinetic modelling demonstrating that the same, uniform weight-based dosing currently applied to every neonate fails to account for gestational-age-specific metabolic differences or altered elimination in the setting of renal impairment.

This does not mean caffeine should be reflexively, permanently discontinued — this same medication carries genuine, established benefit for apnoea of prematurity and bronchopulmonary dysplasia prevention — but rather that individualised dosing and careful monitoring represent the correct, current approach in this specific circumstance.

This directly models this book's own repeated theme: a single medication can carry both genuine, established benefit and a genuine, current safety signal simultaneously, requiring active, individualised clinical judgment rather than an all-or-nothing response.

Why the other options are wrong

A. A genuine, established relationship exists, as detailed in the correct answer, not an absence of relationship.

C. Reflexive, permanent discontinuation is not the correct approach; individualised dosing and monitoring is, given this medication's genuine benefit.

D. Current, uniform dosing does not yet account for these factors; this represents an active area of ongoing research and reconsideration.

E. This infant's own current renal status carries direct, genuine relevance to informing this medication's own dosing going forward.

Board Alert A genuinely current safety signal links early caffeine citrate to acute kidney injury risk. Separately, current pharmacokinetic modelling shows uniform dosing fails to account for gestational-age-specific metabolism or renal impairment.

Question 7

A term infant presents on day 4 of life with significant hypotonia and respiratory distress. The clinical team initially suspects a primary neuromuscular disorder. Rapid genome sequencing is obtained and returns within 36 hours, identifying a pathogenic variant confirming a diagnosis of Pompe disease. Which of the following best describes the most important clinical implication of this specific finding?

A. This diagnosis carries no genuine, specific treatment implication, and this infant's management would be unaffected by this specific result

B. This rapid, correct diagnosis directly enables early initiation of a specific, targeted treatment — enzyme replacement therapy — with genuine, significant potential to improve this infant's own eventual outcome, illustrating the direct, practical value of rapid genomic diagnosis when a targeted therapy genuinely exists

C. This specific diagnosis should prompt immediate discontinuation of all supportive respiratory care, since no meaningful treatment exists for this condition

D. Rapid genome sequencing carries no genuine advantage over traditional, sequential genetic testing in this specific clinical circumstance

E. This infant's hypotonia and respiratory distress are entirely unrelated to this newly identified genetic diagnosis

Answer: B. **This rapid, correct diagnosis directly enables early enzyme replacement therapy, genuinely improving this infant's outcome — illustrating rapid genomic diagnosis's direct, practical value precisely when a targeted therapy exists.**

This vignette directly restates one of this book's own most important, current diagnostic advances: rapid genome sequencing achieving diagnostic turnaround within 24 to 72 hours, with a specific, genuinely moving case example of exactly this presentation — hypotonia and respiratory distress initially suspected to be a primary neuromuscular disorder, ultimately identified as Pompe disease.

This diagnosis's own clinical significance lies specifically in its direct connection to available, targeted treatment: enzyme replacement therapy for Pompe disease, a specific, genuinely serious lysosomal storage disorder, directly benefits from early initiation, making rapid diagnosis genuinely, clinically consequential rather than merely academically interesting.

This illustrates this book's own repeated theme that a genuinely rapid, correct genetic diagnosis can directly translate into life-changing treatment specifically when a targeted therapy genuinely exists for the condition identified — the central, practical argument for rapid sequencing's own current, expanding role in critical neonatal care.

Why the other options are wrong

A. This diagnosis carries a direct, significant treatment implication, as detailed in the correct answer.

C. This condition has a specific, genuine treatment option; supportive care should continue alongside targeted therapy, not be discontinued.

D. Rapid sequencing's genuinely faster turnaround carries direct, practical advantage in this time-sensitive circumstance.

E. This infant's presentation is directly, mechanistically explained by this newly identified diagnosis.

Board Alert Rapid genome sequencing's clinical value is most dramatic when it identifies a treatable condition — Pompe disease directly connects rapid diagnosis to early, life-changing enzyme replacement therapy.

Question 8

A term infant is born to a mother with well-documented type 1 diabetes and demonstrates significant hypoglycaemia, plethora, and cardiomegaly on the first day of life. Which of the following best explains the underlying mechanism connecting this infant's maternal history to this specific clinical presentation?

A. This infant's presentation is entirely coincidental and unrelated to the maternal diabetic history

B. Sustained maternal hyperglycaemia drives fetal hyperinsulinaemia, which directly produces macrosomia, organomegaly including cardiomegaly, and, following delivery and the sudden loss of maternal glucose supply, significant hypoglycaemia as fetal insulin secretion remains transiently elevated

C. This infant's hypoglycaemia reflects a primary pancreatic insufficiency entirely unrelated to maternal glucose exposure

D. Cardiomegaly in this specific context reflects a primary, unrelated structural cardiac malformation rather than a connected, metabolic consequence

E. Maternal diabetes carries no established relationship to neonatal glucose homeostasis of any kind

Answer: B. **Sustained maternal hyperglycaemia drives fetal hyperinsulinaemia, directly producing macrosomia and organomegaly, with significant postnatal hypoglycaemia reflecting transiently persistent fetal insulin secretion after the sudden loss of maternal glucose supply.**

This is the classic infant of a diabetic mother presentation, and this book's own repeated cross-chapter theme connects this single, underlying mechanism — fetal hyperinsulinaemia driven by sustained maternal hyperglycaemia — to each of this infant's specific clinical findings together.

Fetal hyperinsulinaemia directly produces macrosomia and organomegaly, including cardiomegaly, through insulin's own genuine, direct growth-promoting effect on fetal tissue, while plethora reflects connected, elevated haematocrit.

Following delivery, the sudden, complete loss of maternal glucose supply combined with this infant's own transiently, still-elevated insulin secretion directly produces significant, characteristic hypoglycaemia, illustrating this book's repeated demonstration that one connected, underlying mechanism explains an entire, characteristic cluster of findings.

Why the other options are wrong

A. This presentation is directly, mechanistically connected to the maternal diabetic history, not coincidental.

C. This hypoglycaemia reflects transient hyperinsulinism secondary to maternal hyperglycaemia, not primary pancreatic insufficiency.

D. This cardiomegaly reflects a connected, metabolic consequence of fetal hyperinsulinaemia, not an unrelated structural malformation.

E. A direct, well-established relationship exists between maternal diabetes and neonatal glucose homeostasis, as detailed in the correct answer.

Board Alert Infant of a diabetic mother: sustained maternal hyperglycaemia → fetal hyperinsulinaemia → macrosomia, organomegaly, and cardiomegaly antenatally, then significant hypoglycaemia postnatally as maternal glucose supply is suddenly lost.

Mock Exam 1 — Section A: Foundations | Universal Task 4: Management, Treatment and Prevention

Question 9

A 22-week gestation fetus is diagnosed antenatally with a significant, isolated congenital diaphragmatic hernia. The family meets with a coordinated team including maternal-fetal medicine, neonatology, and paediatric surgery to discuss the full range of care options. Which of the following most accurately reflects the correct, complete approach to this specific counselling conversation?

A. Perinatal palliative care should not be discussed, since this diagnosis is not immediately, universally lethal

B. The family should be presented with the complete, honest spectrum of reasonable options — including perinatal palliative care, pregnancy termination where legally available, and active, full resuscitation and postnatal surgical management — with honest acknowledgement that pulmonary hypoplasia severity, rather than defect size alone, often represents the single most important prognostic determinant

C. Postnatal surgical repair should be scheduled for the first hours of life regardless of this infant's own cardiopulmonary status

D. This family's own values and preferences carry no genuine relevance to this specific counselling conversation

E. Only a single treatment pathway should be presented, determined unilaterally by the surgical team alone

Answer: B. This family deserves the complete, honest spectrum of options — perinatal palliative care, termination where available, and active resuscitation with postnatal repair — alongside honest acknowledgement that pulmonary hypoplasia severity, not defect size, often drives prognosis.

This vignette directly integrates this book's own ethics and surgical content together: perinatal palliative care represents one option among a genuinely complete spectrum a family deserves to see in its entirety, informed consent requiring presentation of every reasonable, ethically acceptable option rather than a single, predetermined pathway.

Correct, complete counselling for congenital diaphragmatic hernia specifically requires honest acknowledgement that pulmonary hypoplasia severity, established throughout this book's own surgical content as connecting directly to foundational lung development physiology, frequently represents the single most important prognostic determinant — more so than the diaphragmatic defect's own physical size alone.

Definitive surgical repair, when active management is genuinely chosen, requires delaying surgery until genuine cardiopulmonary stabilisation has been achieved, not scheduling repair reflexively within the first hours of life regardless of this infant's own physiological status.

Why the other options are wrong

A. Perinatal palliative care represents a genuinely reasonable option that should be discussed regardless of a condition's own specific lethality.

C. Surgical repair should genuinely be delayed until cardiopulmonary stabilisation, not scheduled immediately regardless of status.

D. This family's own values and preferences are genuinely central to this counselling conversation, not irrelevant.

E. A complete, honest spectrum of options should genuinely be presented, not a single, unilaterally determined pathway.

Board Alert Congenital diaphragmatic hernia counselling requires the complete spectrum of options and honest acknowledgement that pulmonary hypoplasia severity, not defect size alone, frequently drives prognosis.

Mock Exam 1 — Section B: Organ Systems | Universal Task 4: Management, Treatment and Prevention

Question 10

A 26-week gestation infant develops progressive respiratory distress on day 2 of life with a chest radiograph showing a diffuse, fine granular pattern with air bronchograms. The infant is intubated and given exogenous surfactant. Six hours later, oxygen requirement has improved substantially but the infant now demonstrates a widened pulse pressure, a hyperdynamic precordium, and a systolic murmur. Which of the following is the most likely explanation for this new finding?

A. This represents a new, unrelated congenital cardiac malformation coincidentally presenting at this time

B. The rapid fall in pulmonary vascular resistance following surfactant-mediated improvement in oxygenation has unmasked a haemodynamically significant patent ductus arteriosus, now shunting left-to-right

C. This represents surfactant-induced pulmonary haemorrhage requiring immediate cessation of all respiratory support

D. This finding is entirely unrelated to this infant's own recent surfactant administration or respiratory improvement

E. This represents a normal, expected finding requiring no further evaluation of any kind

Answer: B. Improved oxygenation after surfactant directly lowers pulmonary vascular resistance, unmasking a haemodynamically significant, left-to-right shunting patent ductus arteriosus — explaining the new widened pulse pressure, hyperdynamic precordium, and murmur.

This vignette directly tests the connected physiology this book establishes repeatedly: a widened pulse pressure and hyperdynamic precordium following respiratory improvement represent the classic, connected presentation of a haemodynamically significant patent ductus arteriosus, not a coincidental, new finding.

The mechanism is directly physiological: as surfactant improves oxygenation and lung compliance, pulmonary vascular resistance falls further, and once pulmonary pressure drops below systemic pressure, ductal flow reverses to left-to-right, unmasking a shunt that may have been clinically silent while pulmonary pressures remained elevated.

This connection between respiratory improvement and ductal unmasking represents exactly the kind of cross-system reasoning this book has modelled throughout — recognising that a single, underlying physiological principle explains an apparently new, but genuinely connected, clinical finding.

Why the other options are wrong

A. This presentation directly, physiologically connects to this infant's own recent respiratory course, not a coincidental, new malformation.

C. Pulmonary haemorrhage would not typically produce this specific combination of widened pulse pressure and hyperdynamic precordium.

D. This finding is directly, mechanistically connected to this infant's own recent surfactant administration and improved oxygenation.

E. This finding requires active evaluation and management, not passive observation as an expected, normal finding.

Board Alert Improved oxygenation after surfactant lowers pulmonary vascular resistance, frequently unmasking a haemodynamically significant PDA as pulmonary pressure falls below systemic pressure and shunt direction reverses to left-to-right.

Mock Exam 1 — Section B: Organ Systems | Universal Task 3: Diagnosis, Testing and Monitoring

Question 11

A 28-week gestation infant on day 12 of life develops new-onset apnoea, temperature instability, and feeding intolerance. Abdominal radiography shows pneumatosis intestinalis. Laboratory studies reveal thrombocytopenia and metabolic acidosis. Which of the following findings, if present, would represent the single absolute indication for immediate surgical intervention?

A. Thrombocytopenia alone, regardless of any other specific finding

B. Pneumoperitoneum on abdominal radiography, representing radiological evidence of bowel perforation

C. Metabolic acidosis alone, regardless of any other specific finding

D. Feeding intolerance alone, without any further, connected finding

E. Temperature instability alone, without any further, connected finding

Answer: B. **Pneumoperitoneum — radiological evidence of free intraperitoneal air directly indicating bowel perforation — is the sole absolute indication for immediate surgical intervention in necrotising enterocolitis, distinct from every other finding in this vignette.**

This vignette directly tests this book's own repeated theme regarding necrotising enterocolitis: genuinely current systematic review evidence has identified pneumoperitoneum as the sole absolute indication for immediate surgical intervention, standing apart from an otherwise genuinely uncertain surgical decision-making landscape.

Every other finding in this vignette — thrombocytopenia, metabolic acidosis, feeding intolerance, temperature instability, and pneumatosis intestinalis itself — represents a genuinely important, but non-absolute, indicator requiring integrated, dynamic clinical assessment, since no universally validated threshold exists for identifying an infant definitively failing medical management short of this single, unambiguous radiological finding.

This distinction carries direct, practical significance: correctly recognising which specific finding demands immediate, urgent surgical involvement, as opposed to continued, structured medical management with close monitoring, directly determines the appropriate speed and certainty of this infant's own next step in care.

Why the other options are wrong

A. Thrombocytopenia alone does not represent the single, absolute surgical indication described in the correct answer.

C. Metabolic acidosis alone does not represent the single, absolute surgical indication described in the correct answer.

D. Feeding intolerance alone does not represent the single, absolute surgical indication described in the correct answer.

E. Temperature instability alone does not represent the single, absolute surgical indication described in the correct answer.

> **Board Alert** Pneumoperitoneum is the sole absolute indication for immediate surgery in necrotising enterocolitis — every other finding requires integrated, dynamic clinical judgment within a genuinely uncertain decision-making landscape.

Question 12

A term infant develops significant jaundice on day 3 of life. Total bilirubin is markedly elevated, with a direct fraction under 10 per cent of the total. Maternal and infant blood types are O-positive and A-positive respectively. Direct antiglobulin testing is positive. Which of the following best explains this specific presentation?

A. This presentation reflects biliary atresia, requiring urgent surgical evaluation

B. This presentation reflects ABO incompatibility hemolytic disease, in which maternal anti-A antibodies cross the placenta and cause ongoing hemolysis of this infant's own A-positive red blood cells, directly explaining both the significant indirect hyperbilirubinaemia and the positive direct antiglobulin test

C. This presentation reflects a primary hepatic conjugation defect entirely unrelated to blood type incompatibility

D. This specific combination of maternal and infant blood type carries no established relationship to neonatal jaundice of any kind

E. A positive direct antiglobulin test in this context indicates a laboratory error requiring immediate repeat testing before any further action

> **Answer: B. This is classic ABO incompatibility hemolytic disease: maternal anti-A antibodies cross the placenta and hemolyse this A-positive infant's red blood cells, directly explaining both the significant indirect hyperbilirubinaemia and the positive direct antiglobulin test together.**
>
> This vignette presents the classic combination for ABO incompatibility: an O-positive mother, whose serum naturally contains anti-A and anti-B antibodies capable of crossing the placenta, and an A-positive infant, whose red blood cells become the target of ongoing, maternal antibody-mediated hemolysis.
>
> The predominantly indirect hyperbilirubinaemia (direct fraction under 10 per

cent) directly reflects this ongoing hemolytic process, since unconjugated bilirubin is produced faster than the neonatal liver's own limited conjugation capacity can process, while the positive direct antiglobulin test directly confirms antibody coating of this infant's own red blood cells.

This connected reasoning — recognising a single, underlying immunologic mechanism explaining both the specific pattern of hyperbilirubinaemia and the specific laboratory confirmation together — represents exactly the kind of mechanism-first diagnostic reasoning this book has modelled throughout.

Why the other options are wrong

A. Biliary atresia would present with a predominantly direct, not indirect, hyperbilirubinaemia; this presentation does not fit that pattern.

C. This presentation is directly explained by hemolysis, not a primary, unrelated hepatic conjugation defect.

D. This specific blood type combination carries a direct, well-established relationship to ABO incompatibility hemolytic disease.

E. This positive result directly confirms the correct diagnosis; it does not indicate a laboratory error in this specific clinical context.

Board Alert ABO incompatibility: O-positive mother, A- or B-positive infant, positive direct antiglobulin test, and predominantly indirect hyperbilirubinaemia reflect ongoing, antibody-mediated hemolysis.

Question 13

A 32-week gestation infant with confirmed hypoxic-ischaemic encephalopathy is being considered for therapeutic hypothermia. Which of the following most accurately reflects current, correct practice regarding this specific intervention?

A. Therapeutic hypothermia is equally, well-established and appropriate for this specific gestational age, identical to a term infant

B. Therapeutic hypothermia's own evidence base is most robustly established in the term and late-preterm infant, and its application at 32 weeks gestation requires careful, individualised consideration given more limited evidence in this specific, more preterm population

C. Therapeutic hypothermia carries no established relationship to hypoxic-ischaemic encephalopathy of any kind

D. This intervention should never be considered in any infant born before 37 weeks gestation, regardless of clinical circumstance

E. Gestational age carries no genuine relevance to correctly considering this specific intervention

Answer: B. Therapeutic hypothermia's evidence base is most robustly established in term and late-preterm infants; applying it at 32 weeks requires careful, individualised consideration given the comparatively limited evidence in this more preterm population.

This vignette tests honest, careful attention to the specific boundaries of an established evidence base, directly reflecting this book's own repeated theme of honest evidence treatment rather than uncritical extension of a therapy beyond its own, most robustly studied population.

The foundational, large-scale randomised trials establishing therapeutic hypothermia's own benefit for hypoxic-ischaemic encephalopathy predominantly enrolled term and late-preterm infants, meaning this same intervention's own application at 32 weeks gestation requires genuinely careful, individualised clinical judgment rather than automatic extension of this evidence.

This does not mean the intervention is inappropriate at this gestational age, but rather that correct, honest practice requires actively acknowledging this specific evidence limitation, weighing this infant's own individual circumstance, and involving experienced, specialised clinical judgment in this specific decision.

Why the other options are wrong

A. This evidence base is most robustly established in the term and late-preterm infant, not equally established across every gestational age.

C. This intervention has a direct, well-established relationship to this specific condition in the appropriate population.

D. A rigid, universal exclusion below 37 weeks is not the correct, complete description of current, careful practice.

E. Gestational age carries direct, genuine relevance to correctly considering this specific intervention, as detailed in the correct answer.

Board Alert Therapeutic hypothermia's evidence base is most robust in term and late-preterm infants; application in the more preterm population requires careful, individualised, honestly evidence-limited consideration.

Question 14

A 27-week gestation infant develops a grade III intraventricular haemorrhage on cranial ultrasound performed on day 5 of life. A blood gas obtained on day 1 of life had shown a significant metabolic acidosis with a normal PCO2. Which of the following best explains the specific, connected relevance of this earlier blood gas finding?

A. This earlier finding has no established relationship to this infant's own subsequent intraventricular haemorrhage of any kind

B. Genuinely current research has specifically demonstrated that metabolic acidosis, rather than hypocapnia or hypercapnia specifically, occurring within the first 72 hours of life carries a specific, established association with significant intraventricular haemorrhage, directly connecting this earlier finding to this infant's own subsequent diagnosis

C. Only hypercapnia, not metabolic acidosis, carries any established relationship to intraventricular haemorrhage risk

D. This earlier blood gas finding should have been entirely disregarded, since acid-base status carries no genuine relevance to neurological outcome

E. This specific connection represents an isolated, uncommon finding with no genuine, current research basis of any kind

Answer: B. **Genuinely current research demonstrates that metabolic acidosis specifically, not hypocapnia or hypercapnia, occurring within the first 72 hours of life carries an established association with significant intraventricular haemorrhage — directly connecting this earlier finding to this infant's diagnosis.**

This vignette directly tests a genuinely important, current distinction this book establishes throughout its own acid-base content: it is specifically metabolic acidosis, rather than hypocapnia or hypercapnia, occurring within the first 72 hours of life that carries the established, specific association with significant intraventricular haemorrhage.

This reflects a genuinely important, current research finding directly relevant to correctly calibrating clinical concern — recognising that not every acid-base disturbance carries identical, connected neurological risk, and that correctly distinguishing between genuinely different categories of disturbance directly informs the appropriate degree of vigilance a given finding warrants.

This connected reasoning directly models this book's own repeated demonstration that a specific, early laboratory finding can carry genuine, connected relevance to a later, more serious diagnosis, reinforcing the value of correctly interpreting and remembering earlier clinical data as a case unfolds.

Why the other options are wrong

A. A direct, established relationship exists between this earlier finding and this infant's outcome, as detailed in the correct answer.

C. This reverses the correct relationship; metabolic acidosis, not hypercapnia specifically, carries this specific, established association.

D. This earlier finding carries direct, genuine relevance to neurological outcome, as detailed in the correct answer.

E. This specific connection has direct, genuine basis in current, published research, as detailed in the correct answer.

Board Alert Metabolic acidosis, specifically, occurring within the first 72 hours of life carries an established, current association with significant intraventricular haemorrhage — distinct from hypocapnia or hypercapnia.

Mock Exam 1 — Section B: Organ Systems | Universal Task 4: Management, Treatment and Prevention

Question 15

A 25-week gestation, small-for-gestational-age infant is 34 weeks postmenstrual age. A quality improvement initiative at this NICU has introduced structured screening for iron deficiency using reticulocyte haemoglobin content rather than ferritin. Which of the following best explains the specific rationale for this particular screening choice?

A. Reticulocyte haemoglobin content and ferritin are functionally identical markers with no meaningful, clinical distinction between them

B. Reticulocyte haemoglobin content represents a genuinely more sensitive, more reliable marker of early iron deficiency compared with ferritin, since this specific marker directly reflects iron supply currently available for active erythropoiesis, rather than this infant's own broader, potentially less current iron storage status alone

C. Ferritin represents a genuinely more sensitive marker of early iron deficiency compared with reticulocyte haemoglobin content

D. Neither of these two specific markers carries any genuine, meaningful relevance to correctly screening for iron deficiency in this specific population

E. This specific screening choice has no established basis in any genuinely current quality improvement literature

Answer: B. Reticulocyte haemoglobin content represents a genuinely more sensitive marker of early iron deficiency than ferritin, since it directly reflects iron currently available for active erythropoiesis rather than broader, potentially less current storage status.

This vignette directly tests this book's own genuinely current care systems and quality improvement content: a genuinely current, October 2025 quality improvement initiative specifically selected reticulocyte haemoglobin content over ferritin as its own central screening tool for iron deficiency in the preterm and small-for-gestational-age population.

This specific technical rationale directly explains this choice: reticulocyte haemoglobin content genuinely, directly reflects iron supply currently available for active, ongoing erythropoiesis, providing a more genuinely current picture than ferritin, which reflects broader, potentially less current iron storage status alone.

This same screening initiative carries genuine, connected relevance to neuroprotection, since iron carries genuine, established importance for normal, healthy neurodevelopment — directly connecting a specific haematological screening choice to this infant's own broader, longer-term developmental outcome.

Why the other options are wrong

A. These represent genuinely distinct, non-identical markers with a meaningful, clinical distinction, as detailed in the correct answer.

C. This reverses the correct relationship; reticulocyte haemoglobin content, not ferritin, represents the more sensitive, early marker.

D. Both of these specific markers carry genuine, established relevance to iron deficiency screening, though with differing reliability.

E. This specific screening choice has direct, genuine basis in current, recently published quality improvement literature.

> **Board Alert** Reticulocyte haemoglobin content is a more sensitive marker of early iron deficiency than ferritin, directly reflecting current iron supply for active erythropoiesis rather than broader storage status.

Question 16

A term infant born to a mother with untreated syphilis diagnosed late in the third trimester presents with hepatosplenomegaly, a diffuse maculopapular rash involving the palms and soles, and long bone radiographs showing metaphyseal irregularities. Which of the following best reflects the correct, immediate next step in this infant's evaluation and management?

A. No further evaluation is required, since this presentation is not concerning for any specific, treatable congenital infection

B. This infant's presentation is highly consistent with congenital syphilis, and evaluation should include nontreponemal and treponemal serologic testing on this infant's own serum, along with cerebrospinal fluid analysis, with treatment initiated using intravenous penicillin

C. This presentation should prompt immediate, empiric antifungal therapy rather than any antibacterial treatment

D. Maternal treatment history carries no genuine relevance to correctly evaluating this specific infant

E. This infant's rash and bony findings are unrelated to one another and should be investigated as entirely separate, unconnected clinical problems

> **Answer: B. This presentation — hepatosplenomegaly, a palmar-plantar rash, and metaphyseal irregularities — is highly consistent with congenital syphilis, requiring serologic testing, CSF analysis, and treatment with intravenous penicillin.**
>
> This vignette presents the classic triad of congenital syphilis: hepatosplenomegaly, a characteristic maculopapular rash specifically involving the palms and soles, and metaphyseal irregularities on long bone radiography, occurring in the setting of untreated, late-diagnosed maternal infection.
>
> Correct evaluation directly requires both nontreponemal and treponemal serologic testing on this infant's own serum (rather than cord blood alone,

given the risk of false-positive results from passive maternal antibody transfer), together with cerebrospinal fluid analysis to evaluate for neurosyphilis, since this same evaluation directly informs both diagnosis confirmation and appropriate treatment duration.

Intravenous penicillin represents the correct, established treatment for confirmed or highly probable congenital syphilis, reflecting this book's own repeated theme that correctly, precisely recognising a specific, connected clinical pattern directly informs the appropriate, targeted evaluation and treatment a given infant genuinely requires.

Why the other options are wrong

A. This presentation is genuinely concerning for a specific, treatable congenital infection requiring active evaluation.

C. This presentation is consistent with congenital syphilis, a bacterial infection, not requiring empiric antifungal therapy.

D. Maternal treatment history carries direct, essential relevance to correctly evaluating this infant's own risk and presentation.

E. These findings are directly, mechanistically connected as part of a single, characteristic congenital infection presentation.

Board Alert Congenital syphilis: hepatosplenomegaly, palmar-plantar rash, and metaphyseal irregularities. Evaluate with infant serum serology and CSF analysis; treat with intravenous penicillin.

Question 17

A 29-week gestation infant is 3 weeks old and has been advancing on enteral feeds. The clinical team is discussing whether to add human milk fortifier. Which of the following best reflects the correct, evidence-based rationale for this specific intervention in this population?

A. Human milk alone, without fortification, reliably provides entirely sufficient protein, calcium, and phosphorus to meet this specific population's own elevated nutritional requirements

B. Human milk fortification is generally required to meet the elevated protein, calcium, phosphorus, and caloric requirements of the preterm infant, since unfortified human milk alone typically does not provide sufficient quantities of these specific nutrients to support this population's own accelerated growth requirements

C. Fortification carries no genuine relationship to this population's own bone mineralisation or growth of any kind

D. Fortification should never be added to human milk under any specific circumstance, given genuine, universal safety concerns

E. This infant's specific gestational age carries no genuine relevance to correctly determining nutritional requirements

Answer: B. **Human milk fortification is generally required to meet the preterm infant's elevated protein, calcium, phosphorus, and caloric requirements, since unfortified human milk alone typically does not provide sufficient quantities of these nutrients for this population's accelerated growth needs.**

This vignette directly tests this book's own extensive nutrition content: the preterm infant's own genuinely elevated nutritional requirements, reflecting this population's need to approximate the accelerated growth rate of the third trimester extrauterinely, generally exceed what unfortified human milk alone can reliably provide.

Human milk fortification specifically addresses protein, calcium, phosphorus, and caloric density, directly supporting both this population's own overall growth and, particularly, appropriate bone mineralisation, given this same population's own genuine, elevated risk of metabolic bone disease of prematurity.

This reflects this book's own repeated theme that correctly, individually tailoring nutritional support to this population's own genuinely distinctive requirements, rather than assuming unfortified human milk alone is universally sufficient, directly supports optimal growth and connected, longer-term outcome.

Why the other options are wrong

A. Unfortified human milk alone typically does not provide sufficient quantities of these specific nutrients for this population.

C. A direct, established relationship exists between fortification and bone mineralisation and growth, as detailed in the correct answer.

D. Fortification is generally appropriate and beneficial in this population, not universally contraindicated.

E. This infant's own gestational age carries direct, genuine relevance to determining these requirements, as detailed in the correct answer.

Board Alert Human milk fortification is generally required in the preterm infant to meet elevated protein, calcium, phosphorus, and caloric requirements that unfortified human milk alone typically cannot provide.

Question 18

A term infant develops significant, bilious emesis on day 2 of life with progressive abdominal distension, having never passed meconium despite appearing otherwise well at birth. Which of the following represents the most appropriate, immediate next step in evaluation?

A. Reassurance and continued observation alone, since bilious emesis in a term infant rarely reflects a time-critical surgical circumstance

B. Urgent evaluation for intestinal malrotation with volvulus, a genuinely emergent, time-critical surgical condition, given this infant's specific presentation of significant, bilious emesis

C. Immediate initiation of oral rehydration alone, without any further, specific diagnostic evaluation

D. This presentation should be managed exclusively as simple constipation, without any further, urgent evaluation

E. Bilious emesis in this specific clinical context carries no genuine, particular urgency of any kind

Answer: B. Significant, bilious emesis specifically demands urgent evaluation for intestinal malrotation with volvulus — a genuinely emergent, time-critical surgical condition threatening the entire mesenteric blood supply, not routine observation.

This vignette directly tests this book's own repeated, urgent theme: significant, bilious emesis in a neonate represents a genuinely time-critical warning sign specifically requiring urgent evaluation for intestinal malrotation with volvulus, in which abnormal intestinal rotation creates a narrow mesenteric pedicle around which the bowel can rapidly twist.

This specific twisting can directly, rapidly compromise the entire mesenteric blood supply, threatening genuinely catastrophic, extensive bowel loss within a genuinely narrow, time-critical window — meaning this presentation should never be dismissed as routine, benign feeding intolerance or simple constipation.

The genuine absence of meconium passage further raises this book's own broader differential, including both Hirschsprung disease and an anorectal malformation, but the specific combination with significant, bilious emesis makes urgent, immediate evaluation for this specific, emergent surgical condition the correct, immediate priority.

Why the other options are wrong

A. This specific symptom carries genuine, particular urgency in this context, not warranting reassurance and observation alone.

C. Urgent, specific diagnostic evaluation, not oral rehydration alone, represents the correct, immediate priority.

D. This presentation warrants active, urgent evaluation for a genuinely serious surgical condition, not management as simple constipation.

E. This specific symptom carries genuine, particular, time-critical urgency, as detailed in the correct answer.

Board Alert Bilious emesis in a neonate demands urgent evaluation for intestinal malrotation with volvulus — a genuinely emergent, time-critical surgical condition threatening the entire mesenteric blood supply.

Mock Exam 1 — Section B: Organ Systems | Universal Task 4: Management, Treatment and Prevention

Question 19

A 33-week gestation infant develops respiratory distress shortly after birth. A chest radiograph shows a coarse, streaky infiltrate pattern with fluid in the interlobar fissures, and symptoms substantially improve by 24 hours of life without specific treatment. Which of the following best explains the connected, underlying mechanism for both this infant's presentation and its own genuinely favourable, self-limited course?

A. This presentation reflects a primary surfactant deficiency requiring exogenous surfactant administration

B. This presentation reflects transient tachypnoea of the newborn, in which delayed clearance of fetal lung fluid, connecting to reduced catecholamine-mediated active fluid clearance in the absence of labour, produces this characteristic pattern, with genuine, spontaneous resolution occurring as this same fluid is gradually, physiologically reabsorbed

C. This presentation reflects a significant congenital pneumonia requiring immediate, empiric antibiotic therapy

D. This infant's clinical improvement is entirely unrelated to any specific, underlying physiological mechanism

E. This presentation reflects a significant congenital cardiac malformation requiring immediate surgical evaluation

Answer: B. This is transient tachypnoea of the newborn — delayed fetal lung fluid clearance, particularly given reduced catecholamine-mediated active clearance without labour — with genuine, spontaneous resolution as this fluid is gradually, physiologically reabsorbed.

This vignette presents the classic pattern of transient tachypnoea of the newborn: a coarse, streaky infiltrate with fluid visible in the interlobar fissures, occurring in a late-preterm infant, with genuinely favourable, self-limited resolution within 24 to 72 hours — a pattern genuinely distinct from surfactant deficiency or pneumonia.

This book's own physiology content directly explains this mechanism: active fetal lung fluid clearance genuinely depends on a coordinated, multi-pathway system, including catecholamine-mediated active cellular reabsorption normally, significantly driven by the physiological stress of active labour.

An infant genuinely lacking this same, significant labour-associated catecholamine surge — whether through caesarean delivery without labour or another connected circumstance — carries genuinely elevated risk of this specific presentation, directly explaining both the presentation itself and its own genuinely favourable, self-limited course as this excess fluid is gradually, physiologically cleared.

Why the other options are wrong

A. This specific radiographic pattern and clinical course are more consistent with delayed fluid clearance than primary surfactant deficiency.

C. This presentation's specific, self-limited course is more consistent with transient tachypnoea than a significant, active infection.

D. This infant's clinical improvement is directly, mechanistically explained by gradual, physiological fluid reabsorption.

E. This presentation is not consistent with a significant structural cardiac malformation requiring surgical intervention.

Board Alert Transient tachypnoea of the newborn reflects delayed fetal lung fluid clearance, connecting to reduced catecholamine-mediated active clearance without labour, with genuine, spontaneous resolution as fluid is gradually reabsorbed.

Mock Exam 1 — Section B: Organ Systems | Universal Task 2: Epidemiology and Risk Assessment

Question 20

A 26-week gestation infant is 6 weeks postnatal age and remains on supplemental oxygen and mechanical ventilation. A chest radiograph shows diffuse, hazy opacification with small, cystic changes. Which of the following best reflects the current, evidence-based understanding of the connected risk factors for this infant's likely diagnosis?

A. This infant's diagnosis is unrelated to any specific, identifiable risk factor, occurring entirely at random

B. Both significant hypocapnia occurring before surfactant therapy and, separately, early metabolic acidosis have each been independently associated with increased risk of this diagnosis, reflecting a genuinely bidirectional and multifactorial risk profile requiring active avoidance of extremes in both directions

C. Only hypercapnia, and no other specific acid-base disturbance, carries any established relationship to this specific diagnosis

D. This infant's specific gestational age carries no genuine relevance to this specific diagnosis's own underlying risk profile

E. Mechanical ventilation duration carries no genuine, established relationship to this specific diagnosis of any kind

Answer: B. **Both significant hypocapnia before surfactant therapy and early metabolic acidosis have each been independently associated with increased bronchopulmonary dysplasia risk — a genuinely bidirectional, multifactorial risk profile requiring avoidance of extremes in both directions.**

This vignette presents evolving bronchopulmonary dysplasia, and this book's own repeated, bidirectional risk theme directly applies: significant hypocapnia occurring before surfactant therapy has itself been associated with increased risk, established through historical research, while separately, genuinely current 2024 and 2025 research has demonstrated an association between early metabolic acidosis and this same diagnosis.

This reflects this book's own repeated theme that safe, correctly calibrated ventilator and acid-base management requires actively avoiding excess in either direction — neither excessive hypocapnia nor significant metabolic acidosis represents a genuinely safe extreme, each independently carrying connected, elevated risk.

This connected, multifactorial risk profile directly reinforces why this book has emphasised structured, careful acid-base and ventilator management throughout its own foundational content, rather than focusing on carbon dioxide management alone in isolation from this infant's own broader, connected metabolic status.

Why the other options are wrong

A. Specific, identifiable, connected risk factors exist, as detailed in the correct answer, not entirely random occurrence.

C. Both hypocapnia and metabolic acidosis, not exclusively hypercapnia, carry established relationships to this specific diagnosis.

D. This infant's gestational age carries direct, established relevance to this diagnosis's own risk profile.

E. A direct, established relationship exists between ventilation duration and this specific diagnosis's own risk.

Board Alert Bronchopulmonary dysplasia risk is genuinely bidirectional and multifactorial: significant hypocapnia before surfactant therapy and early metabolic acidosis have each been independently associated with increased risk.

Mock Exam 1 — Section B: Organ Systems | Universal Task 4: Management, Treatment and Prevention

Question 21

A 30-week gestation infant develops signs of significant sepsis on day 10 of life, including temperature instability and increased apnoea. Blood culture eventually grows a coagulase-negative Staphylococcus species. Which of the following best reflects the correct, current approach to interpreting this specific culture result?

A. Every positive blood culture growing coagulase-negative Staphylococcus should automatically be dismissed as a contaminant, regardless of this infant's own clinical presentation

B. Correctly interpreting this specific result requires active, integrated clinical correlation, since coagulase-negative Staphylococcus can represent either a genuine, significant pathogen, particularly in the presence of an indwelling central line, or a contaminant, meaning this infant's own clinical presentation and additional laboratory findings must be actively considered together rather than the culture result interpreted in complete isolation

C. This specific organism can never represent a genuine, clinically significant pathogen in the neonatal population

D. This infant's own clinical presentation carries no genuine relevance to correctly interpreting this specific culture result

E. This specific result should be interpreted identically regardless of whether this infant has an indwelling central venous catheter

Answer: B. **Correctly interpreting a coagulase-negative Staphylococcus culture requires active clinical correlation, since this organism can represent either a genuine pathogen — particularly with an indwelling line — or a contaminant, never interpreted in isolation from this infant's presentation.**

This vignette directly tests this book's own established infectious disease content: coagulase-negative Staphylococcus occupies a genuinely important, nuanced diagnostic category, capable of representing either a genuine, clinically significant pathogen or a contaminant, depending on this infant's own specific, connected clinical circumstance.

An indwelling central venous catheter carries direct, established relevance to this specific interpretation, given this organism's own genuine propensity for line-associated infection, meaning this infant's own line status directly informs the appropriate degree of clinical concern this specific result warrants.

This infant's own significant, connected clinical presentation — temperature instability and increased apnoea — directly supports active, genuine clinical concern rather than reflexive dismissal as a contaminant, reinforcing this book's repeated theme that correctly interpreting a given laboratory result requires active, integrated clinical correlation rather than isolated, formulaic interpretation.

Why the other options are wrong

A. Reflexive dismissal is not the correct approach; active clinical correlation is required, as detailed in the correct answer.

C. This specific organism can genuinely represent a significant pathogen in this population, particularly with an indwelling line.

D. This infant's own clinical presentation carries direct, essential relevance to correctly interpreting this result.

E. Line status carries direct, established relevance to this specific interpretation, as detailed in the correct answer.

Board Alert Coagulase-negative Staphylococcus culture results require active clinical correlation — genuine pathogen versus contaminant — particularly considering indwelling line status and this infant's own connected clinical presentation.

Question 22

A term infant is noted at birth to have ambiguous genitalia. Initial evaluation reveals significant hyponatraemia and hyperkalaemia on day 4 of life. Which of the following represents the most important, immediate diagnostic consideration?

A. This presentation carries no genuine, specific diagnostic urgency of any kind, and evaluation can reasonably be deferred for several weeks

B. Congenital adrenal hyperplasia, specifically 21-hydroxylase deficiency, should be actively, urgently considered, given this infant's combined presentation of ambiguous genitalia and a significant, salt-wasting electrolyte pattern, since this specific diagnosis carries genuine, life-threatening potential if genuinely unrecognised and untreated

C. This specific electrolyte pattern carries no established relationship to ambiguous genitalia of any kind

D. This presentation should be managed exclusively as a primary renal disorder, entirely unrelated to any specific endocrine consideration

E. Ambiguous genitalia in this specific context represents an isolated, cosmetic finding requiring no further, urgent evaluation

Answer: B. Congenital adrenal hyperplasia (21-hydroxylase deficiency) should be urgently considered given ambiguous genitalia combined with a significant, salt-wasting electrolyte pattern — genuinely life-threatening if unrecognised and untreated.

This vignette presents the classic, connected combination for congenital adrenal hyperplasia due to 21-hydroxylase deficiency: ambiguous genitalia, reflecting excess fetal androgen exposure, combined with a significant, salt-wasting electrolyte pattern — hyponatraemia and hyperkalaemia together — reflecting genuine, combined mineralocorticoid and glucocorticoid deficiency.

This specific diagnosis carries genuine, life-threatening urgency, since untreated salt-wasting crisis can rapidly progress to significant hypovolaemic shock, meaning correctly, rapidly recognising this connected presentation and initiating urgent evaluation and treatment carries direct, potentially life-saving importance.

This connected reasoning — recognising that a single, underlying enzymatic deficiency directly explains both the genital and the electrolyte findings together — represents exactly the kind of mechanism-first, urgent diagnostic reasoning this book has modelled throughout its own endocrine and genetics content.

Why the other options are wrong

A. This presentation carries genuine, life-threatening urgency, not reasonably deferred for evaluation.

C. A direct, well-established, mechanistic relationship exists between this specific pattern and this diagnosis.

D. This presentation reflects a significant, connected endocrine disorder, not a primary, unrelated renal disorder.

E. This finding carries direct, urgent diagnostic significance, not representing an isolated, purely cosmetic concern.

Board Alert Ambiguous genitalia with hyponatraemia and hyperkalaemia should urgently raise congenital adrenal hyperplasia (21-hydroxylase deficiency) — a genuinely life-threatening, salt-wasting condition if unrecognised.

Question 23

A 24-week gestation infant is 2 weeks old and has bilateral retinal findings concerning for early retinopathy of prematurity on screening examination. Which of the following best reflects the correct, current approach to this infant's ongoing management?

A. A single, initial screening examination is entirely sufficient, with no further, serial follow-up required regardless of findings

B. Structured, serial ophthalmologic examinations should continue on an appropriate, individualised schedule based on this infant's own specific findings, since retinopathy of prematurity can genuinely progress and serial monitoring directly informs the correct, timely decision regarding treatment when genuinely indicated

C. Treatment should be initiated immediately in every infant with any degree of retinopathy of prematurity, regardless of severity or specific stage

D. This infant's specific gestational age carries no genuine relevance to correctly determining appropriate screening intervals

E. Retinopathy of prematurity never, genuinely progresses once initially identified on screening examination

Answer: B. **Structured, serial ophthalmologic examinations must continue on an individualised schedule, since retinopathy of prematurity can genuinely progress, and this ongoing monitoring directly informs the correct, timely treatment decision when genuinely indicated.**

This vignette tests this book's own established ophthalmology content: retinopathy of prematurity represents a genuinely dynamic, potentially progressive condition requiring structured, serial examination rather than a single, isolated assessment.

This infant's own specific gestational age and current findings directly inform the appropriate, individualised examination interval, since correctly, actively monitoring this same condition's own genuine progression directly determines the correct, timely moment for treatment intervention should this same progression genuinely occur.

This reflects this book's own repeated theme that correctly, safely managing a genuinely dynamic clinical condition requires active, structured, ongoing surveillance, rather than a single, static assessment assumed to remain valid indefinitely.

Why the other options are wrong

A. Serial follow-up is genuinely required, given this condition's own potential for progression, not a single, sufficient examination.

C. Treatment is reserved for specific, defined stages and criteria, not indicated in every degree of retinopathy regardless of severity.

D. This infant's gestational age carries direct, established relevance to determining appropriate screening intervals.

E. This condition can genuinely, actively progress, requiring the structured, serial monitoring detailed in the correct answer.

Board Alert Retinopathy of prematurity requires structured, serial ophthalmologic examination on an individualised schedule, since this condition can genuinely progress, directly informing timely treatment decisions.

Question 24

A 34-week gestation infant develops significant abdominal distension and bilious vomiting on day 1 of life. Abdominal radiography shows a 'double bubble' sign. Genetic testing subsequently confirms trisomy 21. Which of the following best explains the connected relevance of this genetic finding to this infant's specific presentation?

A. This infant's genetic diagnosis is entirely unrelated to this infant's own specific gastrointestinal presentation

B. This radiographic pattern is highly suggestive of duodenal atresia, a specific structural anomaly carrying a genuinely, considerably elevated association with trisomy 21, directly connecting this infant's own confirmed genetic diagnosis to this specific presentation

C. This radiographic pattern reflects jejunoileal atresia, a condition carrying no genuine, established association with trisomy 21

D. Bilious vomiting in this specific context carries no genuine, diagnostic significance of any kind

E. This presentation should be managed without any further, active consideration of this infant's own confirmed genetic status

Answer: B. The 'double bubble' sign is highly suggestive of duodenal atresia, a specific structural anomaly carrying a genuinely, considerably elevated association with trisomy 21, directly connecting this genetic diagnosis to this specific presentation.

This vignette directly tests this book's own repeated, cross-domain connection: the specific, characteristic 'double bubble' radiographic sign directly reflects duodenal atresia, and this book has established throughout that duodenal atresia specifically carries a genuinely, considerably elevated association with trisomy 21.

This connection is genuinely important and location-specific: jejunoileal atresia, by contrast, more typically reflects a genuinely different, specific mechanism — an isolated, in utero vascular accident — carrying no comparable, established chromosomal association, making correct anatomical localisation directly relevant to genetic counselling.

This case directly illustrates this book's own repeated demonstration that correctly, precisely identifying a given structural anomaly's own specific anatomical location and connected genetic association together directly informs both this infant's own immediate surgical management and this same infant's own broader, longer-term diagnostic evaluation.

Why the other options are wrong

A. A direct, well-established, connected relationship exists between this diagnosis and this presentation, as detailed in the correct answer.

C. This specific radiographic pattern reflects duodenal, not jejunoileal, atresia, which carries this specific trisomy 21 association.

D. This specific symptom carries direct, significant diagnostic relevance in this presentation, as detailed in the correct answer.

E. This infant's own confirmed genetic status carries direct, connected relevance to this presentation and its own broader evaluation.

Board Alert The 'double bubble' sign reflects duodenal atresia, which carries a considerably elevated association with trisomy 21 — genuinely distinct from jejunoileal atresia's own connection to an isolated, in utero vascular accident.

Question 25

A 27-week gestation infant is 4 weeks old, remains on parenteral nutrition, and has developed a direct hyperbilirubinaemia with a direct fraction exceeding 20 per cent of the total bilirubin. Which of the following best reflects the most likely underlying explanation for this specific finding?

A. This finding reflects ongoing, physiologic hemolysis unrelated to this infant's own nutritional support

B. This finding is most consistent with parenteral nutrition-associated cholestasis, a genuinely important, connected complication of prolonged parenteral nutrition particularly relevant in the extremely preterm population, warranting active consideration of advancing enteral feeds where genuinely possible

C. This finding carries no genuine, established relationship to this infant's own duration of parenteral nutrition of any kind

D. This finding should be managed identically to a predominantly indirect hyperbilirubinaemia, with no genuine, specific distinction in approach

E. This specific pattern of hyperbilirubinaemia requires no further evaluation of any kind

Answer: B. **A direct fraction exceeding 20 per cent in an infant on prolonged parenteral nutrition is most consistent with parenteral nutrition-associated cholestasis — warranting active consideration of advancing enteral feeds where genuinely possible.**

This vignette directly tests this book's own extensive nutrition content: a predominantly direct hyperbilirubinaemia, rather than an indirect pattern, occurring in the setting of prolonged parenteral nutrition is most consistent with parenteral nutrition-associated cholestasis, a genuinely important, recognised complication particularly relevant in the extremely preterm population requiring extended parenteral support.

This specific finding directly requires a genuinely different diagnostic and management approach compared with indirect hyperbilirubinaemia, since this direct pattern reflects hepatobiliary dysfunction rather than excess bilirubin production, directly informing correct, targeted management.

This same finding directly, practically supports active consideration of advancing enteral feeds where genuinely, clinically possible, since this same, active transition toward enteral nutrition represents a genuinely important, established strategy for both preventing and managing this specific, connected complication.

Why the other options are wrong

A. This specific, direct pattern is more consistent with cholestasis than physiologic hemolysis, which typically produces an indirect pattern.

C. A direct, established relationship exists between parenteral nutrition duration and this specific complication.

D. This direct pattern requires a genuinely different, specific management approach compared with an indirect pattern.

E. This specific finding warrants active evaluation and management, as detailed in the correct answer.

Board Alert A predominantly direct hyperbilirubinaemia in an infant on prolonged parenteral nutrition is most consistent with parenteral nutrition-associated cholestasis, warranting active consideration of advancing enteral feeds.

Question 26

A term infant develops significant respiratory distress within the first hour of life. A chest radiograph shows a scaphoid abdomen with bowel loops visible within the thoracic cavity, and the cardiac silhouette is shifted to the right. Which of the following best reflects the correct, immediate approach to this infant's initial respiratory management?

A. Immediate, vigorous bag-mask ventilation with a face mask represents the correct, preferred approach to this infant's initial respiratory support

B. This infant's presentation is consistent with congenital diaphragmatic hernia, and face mask ventilation should specifically be avoided given the genuine risk of further gastric and bowel distension worsening pulmonary compression, with immediate intubation representing the preferred approach instead

C. This infant's presentation carries no genuine, specific relevance to correctly selecting an appropriate mode of respiratory support

D. This infant should be managed with high-flow nasal cannula alone, without consideration of more advanced, invasive respiratory support

E. The specific position of this infant's cardiac silhouette carries no genuine, diagnostic relevance to this presentation

Answer: B. **This presentation is consistent with congenital diaphragmatic hernia. Face mask ventilation should specifically be avoided, since it risks further gastric and bowel distension worsening pulmonary compression — immediate intubation is preferred instead.**

This vignette presents the classic findings of congenital diaphragmatic hernia: a scaphoid abdomen, bowel loops visible within the thoracic cavity, and mediastinal shift, directly reflecting herniation of abdominal contents into the thorax through the diaphragmatic defect.

This book's own resuscitation content directly establishes a specific, important exception to standard respiratory support: face mask ventilation should specifically be avoided in this exact presentation, since positive pressure delivered through a mask directly risks further inflating the stomach and bowel loops already occupying thoracic space, directly worsening pulmonary compression.

Immediate intubation, rather than mask ventilation, represents the correct, preferred initial approach in this specific, recognisable presentation, directly illustrating this book's own repeated theme that correctly, rapidly recognising a specific, connected clinical pattern directly changes the appropriate, immediate management approach.

Why the other options are wrong

A. Face mask ventilation should specifically be avoided in this presentation, as detailed in the correct answer, not preferred.

C. This presentation carries direct, specific relevance to selecting the correct, appropriate mode of respiratory support.

D. This infant's presentation requires more advanced, definitive respiratory support, not high-flow nasal cannula alone.

E. This specific finding carries direct, diagnostic relevance to this presentation, reflecting mediastinal shift.

Board Alert Congenital diaphragmatic hernia: scaphoid abdomen, thoracic bowel loops, mediastinal shift. Avoid face mask ventilation given risk of worsening gastric and bowel distension; proceed to immediate intubation instead.

Question 27

A 25-week gestation infant is 8 weeks old and undergoes routine cranial ultrasound surveillance, which shows periventricular echolucencies consistent with evolving cystic periventricular leukomalacia. Which of the following best reflects the correct, current understanding of this specific finding's own connected significance?

A. This finding carries no genuine, established relationship to this infant's own longer-term neurodevelopmental outcome of any kind

B. This finding reflects white matter injury carrying genuine, established relevance to this infant's own longer-term neurodevelopmental outcome, including elevated risk of cerebral palsy, supporting the same structured, longer-term neurodevelopmental follow-up this book has established throughout as essential for this population

C. This finding is entirely reversible with no genuine, longer-term consequence of any kind

D. This finding requires no further, structured follow-up of any kind, since periventricular leukomalacia carries no established clinical significance

E. This specific finding is unrelated to this infant's own extreme prematurity or connected, perinatal course

Answer: B. Cystic periventricular leukomalacia reflects white matter injury with genuine, established relevance to longer-term neurodevelopmental outcome, including elevated cerebral palsy risk — supporting structured, longer-term follow-up.

This vignette directly tests this book's own established neurology content: cystic periventricular leukomalacia reflects genuine, significant white matter injury, carrying established, connected relevance to this infant's own longer-term neurodevelopmental trajectory, including a genuinely elevated risk of cerebral palsy and other connected motor and cognitive impairment.

This finding directly supports the same structured, longer-term neurodevelopmental follow-up programme this book has established repeatedly throughout its own content as essential for this high-risk population, extending clinical attention well beyond the acute, immediate neonatal period alone.

This reflects this book's own repeated, cross-chapter theme that a specific, acute radiographic finding frequently carries direct, connected relevance to a considerably longer-term, connected clinical trajectory, reinforcing the genuine importance of coordinated, structured surveillance extending across this infant's own entire, connected developmental journey.

Why the other options are wrong

A. A direct, well-established relationship exists between this finding and longer-term outcome, as detailed in the correct answer.

C. This finding carries genuine, established longer-term consequence, not being entirely reversible without lasting effect.

D. This finding requires structured, longer-term follow-up, given its own established clinical significance.

E. A direct, established relationship exists between this finding and this infant's own extreme prematurity.

Board Alert Cystic periventricular leukomalacia reflects white matter injury with established relevance to longer-term neurodevelopmental outcome, including elevated cerebral palsy risk, supporting structured, longer-term follow-up.

Question 28

A 26-week gestation infant is being supported on extracorporeal membrane oxygenation for confirmed, severe persistent pulmonary hypertension genuinely failing maximal conventional therapy. Which of the following best reflects an important, connected consideration specific to this infant's own extreme prematurity in this specific context?

A. This infant's extreme prematurity carries no genuine, particular relevance to this infant's own candidacy or management on this specific technology

B. This infant's extreme prematurity represents a specific, important relative contraindication to this technology, since this same technology's own required anticoagulation directly compounds this population's own already elevated, established bleeding vulnerability, requiring active, careful weighing of this connected risk against this technology's own genuine, potential benefit

C. Anticoagulation carries no genuine, meaningful relationship to bleeding risk in this specific population

D. Extreme prematurity represents a genuinely favourable, rather than a relatively contraindicated, factor for this specific technology

E. This infant's own gestational age has already been fully, formally excluded as a relevant consideration in current, established candidacy guidelines

Answer: B. **This infant's extreme prematurity represents a specific, important relative contraindication to ECMO, since this technology's required anticoagulation directly compounds this population's already elevated bleeding vulnerability, requiring careful risk-benefit weighing.**

This vignette directly tests this book's own established ECMO content: extreme prematurity and genuinely low birthweight represent specific, important relative contraindications to this technology, connecting directly to this population's own genuinely elevated, established bleeding vulnerability.

This same technology's own genuine, required anticoagulation directly, considerably compounds this already elevated risk, meaning correctly, safely determining candidacy in this specific circumstance requires actively, carefully weighing this connected, genuine risk against this technology's own genuine, potential benefit for this infant's own confirmed, severe condition.

This reflects this book's own repeated theme that a genuinely powerful, potentially life-saving technology still requires active, individualised clinical judgment in this specific, genuinely challenging population, rather than a uniform, reflexive application regardless of this infant's own particular, connected risk profile.

Why the other options are wrong

A. This infant's own extreme prematurity carries direct, particular relevance to candidacy, as detailed in the correct answer.

C. A direct, mechanistic relationship exists between anticoagulation and bleeding risk in this population.

D. This represents a relatively contraindicated, not favourable, factor for this specific technology.

E. Gestational age remains a genuine, active consideration in candidacy determination, as detailed in the correct answer.

Board Alert Extreme prematurity represents a relative contraindication to ECMO, given this technology's required anticoagulation compounding this population's already elevated, established bleeding vulnerability.

Question 29

A term infant born to a mother with poorly controlled hyperthyroidism during pregnancy develops tachycardia, irritability, and poor weight gain in the first week of life. Which of the following best explains this infant's presentation?

A. This presentation is entirely coincidental and unrelated to the maternal thyroid history

B. This presentation is consistent with neonatal Graves disease, reflecting transplacental passage of maternal thyroid-stimulating immunoglobulins, requiring active monitoring and, where genuinely indicated, specific treatment given this condition's own potential for significant, connected cardiovascular complication

C. This presentation reflects primary congenital hypothyroidism, entirely unrelated to the maternal hyperthyroid history

D. Maternal thyroid antibody status carries no genuine relevance to this infant's own presentation of any kind

E. This presentation requires no further, active evaluation or monitoring of any kind

Answer: B. This presentation is consistent with neonatal Graves disease, reflecting transplacental passage of maternal thyroid-stimulating immunoglobulins, requiring active monitoring given this condition's potential for significant cardiovascular complication.

This vignette presents neonatal Graves disease, in which maternal thyroid-stimulating immunoglobulins directly cross the placenta and stimulate this infant's own thyroid gland, producing a transient, but genuinely significant, hyperthyroid state.

This connected mechanism directly explains this infant's own presentation: tachycardia, irritability, and poor weight gain together reflect a genuinely elevated metabolic state, directly mirroring the maternal condition through this same, connected antibody-mediated mechanism.

This condition carries genuine, potential significance for significant cardiovascular complication, including tachyarrhythmia and, in severe cases, cardiac failure, meaning active, structured monitoring and, where genuinely indicated, specific treatment represent the correct, appropriate approach, rather than assuming this presentation will spontaneously, safely resolve without any active clinical attention.

Why the other options are wrong

A. This presentation is directly, mechanistically connected to the maternal thyroid history, not coincidental.

C. This presentation reflects a transient hyperthyroid, not a primary hypothyroid, state, directly connected to the maternal history.

D. Maternal antibody status carries direct, mechanistic relevance to this infant's own presentation.

E. This condition warrants active evaluation and monitoring, given its own potential for significant complication.

Board Alert Neonatal Graves disease reflects transplacental passage of maternal thyroid-stimulating immunoglobulins, producing tachycardia, irritability, and poor weight gain, with genuine potential for significant cardiovascular complication.

Question 30

A 25-week gestation infant, now 3 weeks old, has undergone routine neuroimaging surveillance and been diagnosed with a grade IV intraventricular haemorrhage with periventricular hemorrhagic infarction. The family is meeting with the clinical team to discuss this infant's own ongoing care. Which of the following best reflects the correct, complete approach to this specific conversation?

A. This family should be presented with a single, predetermined care plan without further, genuine discussion

B. This family deserves a genuine, shared decision-making conversation, honestly incorporating this specific finding's own genuine prognostic significance, together with the full range of reasonable options this circumstance may now present, with this same family's own values and preferences genuinely, actively centred throughout

C. This specific finding carries no genuine relevance to this family's own ongoing decision-making regarding this infant's care

D. This conversation should be deferred indefinitely, since this specific finding requires no further, active discussion

E. This family's own preferences carry no genuine relevance to this specific circumstance, which should be determined entirely by the clinical team alone

Answer: B. **This family deserves a genuine, shared decision-making conversation, honestly incorporating this finding's genuine prognostic significance alongside the full range of reasonable options, with this family's own values genuinely centred throughout.**

This vignette directly integrates this book's own neurology and ethics content together: a grade IV intraventricular haemorrhage with periventricular hemorrhagic infarction carries genuine, significant prognostic implication, and this same, honest significance should be genuinely, actively incorporated into a shared decision-making conversation with this family.

This book's own repeated, foundational ethics principle directly applies here: shared decision-making, emphasising genuine partnership, complete transparency, and respect for this family's own genuine values, represents the current, gold-standard approach to this exact kind of genuinely difficult, connected clinical circumstance.

This means this family deserves the full range of reasonable options this circumstance may now present, honestly and completely, with this same family's own values and preferences genuinely, actively centred throughout — precisely the same, connected reasoning this book has modelled throughout its ethics and palliative care content for every genuinely difficult, high-stakes clinical circumstance.

Why the other options are wrong

A. A genuine, shared conversation, not a single, predetermined plan, represents the correct, complete approach.

C. This specific finding carries direct, genuine relevance to this family's own ongoing decision-making.

D. This conversation should genuinely, actively occur, not be deferred indefinitely.

E. This family's own preferences are genuinely, actively central to this circumstance, not excluded from this determination.

Board Alert A significant neurological finding requires genuine, shared decision-making — honest prognostic discussion combined with the full range of reasonable options, with this family's own values genuinely centred throughout.

Question 31

A term infant develops significant, delayed passage of meconium beyond 48 hours of life, with progressive abdominal distension but no bilious emesis. Rectal examination reveals a normal-appearing anus. Which of the following represents the most appropriate next diagnostic step?

A. No further evaluation is required, since delayed meconium passage beyond 48 hours carries no genuine, diagnostic significance

B. Active evaluation for Hirschsprung disease should be pursued, given this infant's specific presentation, since this condition's own underlying mechanism — congenital absence of ganglion cells within a variable segment of distal bowel — directly explains this exact, characteristic clinical pattern

C. This presentation should be managed exclusively as simple constipation, without further, specific diagnostic evaluation

D. This presentation is inconsistent with any specific, recognised neonatal surgical condition

E. A normal-appearing anus on examination definitively excludes every possible cause of this specific presentation

Answer: B. Active evaluation for Hirschsprung disease should be pursued, since congenital absence of ganglion cells within a variable segment of distal bowel directly explains this infant's exact, characteristic pattern of delayed meconium passage and progressive distension.

This vignette directly tests this book's own foundational surgical mechanism: significant, delayed passage of meconium beyond 48 hours of life represents a specific, genuinely important clinical sign directly reflecting the functional obstruction Hirschsprung disease's own underlying mechanism genuinely, mechanistically produces.

Congenital absence of ganglion cells within a specific, variable segment of distal bowel directly prevents this same, affected segment from achieving the normal, coordinated peristaltic relaxation healthy bowel tissue genuinely requires, directly explaining both the delayed meconium passage and the progressive abdominal distension together.

A normal-appearing anus on examination directly helps distinguish this presentation from an anorectal malformation, which typically presents with a genuinely visible, structural abnormality, supporting active, further evaluation specifically for Hirschsprung disease in this exact, connected clinical circumstance.

Why the other options are wrong

A. This presentation carries genuine, significant diagnostic significance, warranting active further evaluation.

C. This presentation warrants active, specific evaluation for a recognised surgical condition, not management as simple constipation alone.

D. This presentation is consistent with a specific, recognised neonatal surgical condition, as detailed in the correct answer.

E. A normal-appearing anus helps distinguish this presentation from an anorectal malformation but does not exclude Hirschsprung disease.

Board Alert Hirschsprung disease reflects congenital absence of ganglion cells within a variable distal bowel segment, directly producing functional obstruction and this characteristic pattern of delayed meconium passage and distension.

Question 32

A 28-week gestation infant has completed a genuinely prolonged, 8-day continuous morphine infusion for postoperative pain management following significant abdominal surgery. The clinical team is now planning discontinuation. Which of the following best reflects the correct, current approach to this specific circumstance?

A. This infusion should be discontinued abruptly, without any genuine, specific concern for connected withdrawal risk

B. This infant's genuinely prolonged infusion duration carries a genuine, significant risk of narcotic withdrawal symptoms upon discontinuation, requiring a genuinely gradual, structured weaning process rather than abrupt cessation

C. Infusion duration carries no genuine, meaningful relationship to withdrawal risk of any kind

D. This infant requires no further, active pain assessment once this infusion has been fully discontinued

E. This specific consideration has no relationship to any established, current clinical guidance

Answer: B. **This infant's genuinely prolonged, 8-day infusion carries a significant risk of narcotic withdrawal symptoms upon discontinuation, requiring a gradual, structured weaning process rather than abrupt cessation.**

This vignette directly tests this book's own established pharmacology content: neonates genuinely treated with a continuous opioid infusion for a genuinely prolonged duration, established as approximately 5 days or considerably longer, are genuinely, significantly more likely to develop specific narcotic withdrawal symptoms once this infusion is genuinely, eventually discontinued.

This infant's own 8-day infusion duration directly exceeds this specific, practical threshold, meaning correctly, safely managing this specific circumstance requires actively, proactively anticipating this specific, connected withdrawal risk, generally through a genuinely gradual, structured weaning process rather than abrupt discontinuation.

This reflects this book's own repeated theme that a specific medication's own genuine, connected risk frequently extends well beyond its own initial administration, requiring active, ongoing clinical attention throughout the entire, genuine duration of treatment and into its own eventual, careful discontinuation.

Why the other options are wrong

A. Genuine, significant withdrawal risk exists, requiring a gradual, structured approach, not abrupt discontinuation.

C. A direct, established relationship exists between infusion duration and withdrawal risk, as detailed in the correct answer.

D. Active, ongoing pain and withdrawal assessment remains genuinely important even following discontinuation.

E. This specific consideration has direct, established basis in current clinical guidance, as detailed in the correct answer.

Board Alert Neonates receiving a continuous opioid infusion for approximately 5 days or longer are significantly more likely to develop narcotic withdrawal symptoms, requiring gradual, structured weaning rather than abrupt discontinuation.

Question 33

A 24-week gestation infant with confirmed, severe persistent pulmonary hypertension, genuinely failing maximal conventional medical therapy at a referring, Level II facility, is being evaluated for extracorporeal membrane oxygenation and transfer. Genuinely current, portable ECMO console technology is available at this same referring facility. Which of the following best reflects the correct, current approach to this specific circumstance?

A. This infant should always, definitively be transported first, with extracorporeal support only ever considered once this infant has physically reached a specialised, Level IV facility

B. Genuinely current technological advances may enable safe cannulation and ECMO initiation at this referring facility before transport actually begins, requiring the specialised, coordinated mobile ECMO team this circumstance directly demands, rather than reflexively assuming transport must always precede this specific technology

C. This infant's specific facility level carries no genuine relevance to correctly planning this infant's own transport and ECMO approach

D. Genuinely current technological advances carry no genuine relevance to correctly planning this specific transport approach

E. This circumstance can be correctly, safely managed by a single, standard transport clinician acting entirely independently

Answer: B. Genuinely current, portable ECMO console technology may enable safe cannulation at this referring facility before transport begins, requiring the specialised, coordinated mobile ECMO team this circumstance demands, rather than assuming transport must always precede this technology.

This vignette directly tests this book's own genuinely current transport and ECMO content: genuinely current technological advances, including a specific, portable ECMO console genuinely certified for ground transport, have directly enabled extracorporeal membrane oxygenation initiation at a genuinely referring centre, even for high-risk transports, rather than exclusively at a specialised centre before subsequent transport.

This means this genuinely current shift directly reflects an important, evolving change in correctly, safely managing the critically ill infant genuinely requiring this technology before this infant can actually, physically reach a specialised centre.

Correctly, safely performing this genuinely complex, combined process directly requires a specialised, mobile ECMO team, this same, specialised team genuinely combining specific technical expertise directly relevant to this technology together with specific, further expertise directly relevant to safe, active interhospital transport.

Why the other options are wrong

A. Genuinely current technology may enable on-site initiation before transport, not requiring transport to always precede this technology.

C. This infant's own facility level carries direct, genuine relevance to planning this specific approach, as detailed in the correct answer.

D. These specific advances carry direct, genuine relevance to planning this transport approach, as detailed in the correct answer.

E. This genuinely complex process requires coordinated, specialised management, not a single clinician acting entirely independently.

Board Alert Genuinely current, portable ECMO console technology can enable safe cannulation at a referring facility before transport, requiring a specialised, coordinated mobile ECMO team combining both extracorporeal and transport expertise.

Question 34

A Level II neonatal intensive care unit, genuinely struggling with a significant, ongoing nursing staff shortage, identifies an opportunity to improve its own current procedural pain management practices, currently well below established benchmarks. Which of the following represents the correct, structured, first step in addressing this specific opportunity?

A. Immediate, broad, systemwide implementation of a new protocol, without any genuine, preceding small-scale trial

B. Formulating a specific, measurable, actionable, realistic, and timely aim, then applying the Plan-Do-Study-Act cycle beginning with a small-scale, initial trial to identify and correct any genuine, unanticipated problem before broader, systemwide implementation

C. This specific improvement opportunity requires no genuine, structured methodology of any kind, relying entirely on informal, individual effort

D. This unit's own genuine staffing constraint carries no genuine relevance to planning this specific improvement initiative

E. Connecting with a broader, coordinated quality improvement network carries no genuine relevance to this specific, single-facility effort

Answer: B. The correct first step is formulating a specific SMART aim, then applying the Plan-Do-Study-Act cycle beginning with a small-scale, initial trial to identify and correct problems before broader, systemwide implementation.

This vignette directly tests this book's own established quality improvement methodology: correctly, effectively structuring a given improvement initiative requires actively, deliberately defining a specific, measurable, actionable, realistic, and timely aim before this same initiative's own subsequent implementation actually begins.

The Plan-Do-Study-Act cycle then directly requires a small-scale, initial trial, since this same, small-scale approach directly allows a given team to identify and correct a genuine, unanticipated problem while this same problem's own actual, practical consequence remains genuinely limited, rather than a single, immediate, broad implementation.

This unit's own honestly acknowledged nursing shortage directly constrains this same initiative's own practical, realistic implementation, meaning correctly, effectively engaging frontline nursing staff and considering connection with a broader, coordinated network, established throughout this book's care systems content, could directly support this same effort despite this genuine, ongoing constraint.

Why the other options are wrong

A. A small-scale, initial trial, not immediate, broad implementation, represents the correct, structured first step.

C. This specific opportunity benefits from structured, established methodology, not informal, individual effort alone.

D. This constraint carries direct, genuine relevance to planning this specific initiative, as detailed in the correct answer.

E. This broader network carries direct, genuine relevance to supporting this specific effort, as detailed in the correct answer.

Board Alert Correct quality improvement methodology begins with a specific SMART aim, then a small-scale Plan-Do-Study-Act trial to identify and correct problems before broader, systemwide implementation.

Question 35

A family receives a significant, life-limiting fetal diagnosis at 22 weeks gestation and meets with the coordinated obstetric and neonatal teams to discuss this pregnancy's own remaining course. Which of the following best reflects the correct, complete, and compassionate approach to this specific conversation?

A. This family should be presented with only the single option the clinical team itself genuinely prefers

B. This family deserves the entire, full spectrum of reasonable options, including perinatal palliative care, pregnancy termination where legally available, and active, full resuscitation and treatment, presented honestly and completely, with this family's own genuine values and final decision-making authority actively centred throughout

C. Perinatal palliative care should not be discussed, since this pathway is inferior to active, full resuscitation in every specific circumstance

D. This family's own genuine values carry no genuine relevance to this specific conversation

E. This conversation should be conducted entirely by a single discipline, without any genuine, coordinated, multidisciplinary involvement

Answer: B. This family deserves the entire, full spectrum of reasonable options — palliative care, termination where available, and active resuscitation — presented honestly and completely, with their own genuine values and final authority centred throughout.

This vignette directly tests this book's own foundational ethics principle: perinatal palliative care represents one, specific option along a genuinely broader spectrum of care, this same spectrum also genuinely including pregnancy termination and full, active neonatal resuscitation and treatment together.

Correctly, completely honouring informed consent requires this family genuinely being presented with this entire, full array of reasonable, ethically acceptable options, rather than a single option presented in isolation or reflecting only the clinical team's own, personal preference.

This same conversation directly requires the same, genuinely coordinated, multidisciplinary involvement this book has established repeatedly throughout — obstetric and neonatal teams together — with this family's own final decision-making authority genuinely, actively honoured throughout this entire, compassionate process.

Why the other options are wrong

A. This family deserves the entire, full spectrum of options, not a single option the team itself genuinely prefers.

C. Perinatal palliative care represents a genuinely reasonable, legitimate option, not an inferior pathway to be excluded from discussion.

D. This family's own genuine values carry direct, essential relevance to this conversation, as detailed in the correct answer.

E. This conversation requires genuine, coordinated, multidisciplinary involvement, not a single discipline acting alone.

Board Alert A family facing a life-limiting fetal diagnosis deserves the complete, honest spectrum of options — palliative care, termination, and active resuscitation — with their own values and final authority centred throughout.

Question 36

A genuinely current, specific randomised controlled trial reports that a new medication significantly reduces a serious neonatal outcome, with a relative risk reduction of 35 per cent and a p-value below 0.05. The baseline risk of this outcome in the control group was 2 per cent. Which of the following best reflects the correct, complete interpretation of this specific finding?

A. This relative risk reduction alone provides an entirely complete, sufficient picture of this medication's own genuine clinical importance

B. This impressive relative risk reduction should be translated into an absolute risk reduction, given this outcome's own genuinely low baseline risk, since a genuinely impressive relative reduction can reflect only a genuinely small, absolute risk reduction when baseline risk is already low, directly informing this medication's own genuine, practical clinical importance through the number needed to treat

C. Statistical significance alone genuinely confirms this same finding's own real, practical clinical importance

D. This specific outcome's own baseline risk carries no genuine relevance to correctly interpreting this reported benefit

E. A p-value below 0.05 eliminates any genuine need for further, critical statistical interpretation of any kind

Answer: B. **This impressive relative risk reduction should be translated into an absolute risk reduction, since a genuinely impressive relative figure can reflect only a small, absolute reduction when baseline risk is already low — directly informing genuine clinical importance through the number needed to treat.**

This vignette directly tests this book's own foundational biostatistics content: absolute risk reduction, the genuine, actual difference in risk between two groups, is genuinely, specifically distinct from relative risk reduction, the genuine, proportional reduction expressed relative to baseline risk.

With a baseline risk of only 2 per cent, a 35 per cent relative reduction translates to an absolute risk reduction of only 0.7 percentage points — directly illustrating this book's own repeated theme that a genuinely impressive, relative figure can reflect only a genuinely small, absolute effect when baseline risk is already low.

Correctly, critically interpreting this specific finding also requires actively distinguishing genuine statistical significance from genuine clinical significance, since a p-value alone confirms only that this result is unlikely to have occurred by chance, not that this same result carries genuine, practical clinical importance — reinforcing this book's repeated theme that critical appraisal requires more than a single, favourable statistic.

Why the other options are wrong

A. This relative figure alone is genuinely insufficient; absolute risk reduction and number needed to treat are also required.

C. Statistical significance alone does not confirm genuine clinical importance, as detailed in the correct answer.

D. This baseline risk carries direct, essential relevance to correctly interpreting this reported benefit, as detailed in the correct answer.

E. Further, critical statistical interpretation remains genuinely necessary, not eliminated by statistical significance alone.

Board Alert A genuinely impressive relative risk reduction can reflect only a small, absolute risk reduction when baseline risk is already low — always translate to absolute risk reduction and number needed to treat for genuine clinical interpretation.

Question 37

A 32-week gestation infant develops a significant, new-onset seizure on day 2 of life. Serum glucose, calcium, and sodium are all within normal range. Cranial ultrasound is unremarkable. Which of the following represents an important, additional diagnostic consideration in this specific circumstance?

A. No further evaluation is required, since normal metabolic studies and cranial ultrasound entirely exclude any further, active diagnostic consideration

B. Active consideration of a specific, underlying inborn error of metabolism remains genuinely important, since normal, routine metabolic studies do not entirely exclude this broader category, and the critical sample principle, correctly timing specific laboratory collection during genuine, active clinical decompensation, carries direct, particular importance in this specific evaluation

C. This infant's presentation carries no genuine relevance to any further, specific metabolic evaluation of any kind

D. Cranial ultrasound findings alone provide an entirely complete, sufficient evaluation for neonatal seizure of any specific etiology

E. This presentation should be managed without any further, active diagnostic evaluation of any kind

Answer: B. Active consideration of an underlying inborn error of metabolism remains genuinely important, since normal, routine

studies do not exclude this broader category — the critical sample principle carries particular importance in this specific evaluation.

This vignette directly tests this book's own established principle: a genuinely important, broader differential for neonatal seizure includes specific, less common causes beyond routine glucose, calcium, and sodium, including an inborn error of metabolism, which routine, standard metabolic studies alone do not entirely exclude.

The critical sample principle, established throughout this book's own endocrine and genetics content, directly extends to this specific circumstance: obtaining specific, relevant laboratory samples at the precise moment of genuine, active clinical decompensation directly provides the most genuinely diagnostic, otherwise fleeting information regarding a specific, underlying metabolic abnormality.

This reflects this book's own repeated theme that a normal, routine evaluation does not necessarily, entirely exclude a further, genuinely important diagnostic category, and that correctly, comprehensively evaluating a genuinely concerning presentation requires active, structured consideration of this broader, connected differential.

Why the other options are wrong

A. Further, active diagnostic consideration remains genuinely important, as detailed in the correct answer.

C. This presentation carries direct, genuine relevance to further metabolic evaluation, as detailed in the correct answer.

D. A normal cranial ultrasound does not provide an entirely complete evaluation for every possible seizure etiology.

E. Further, active diagnostic evaluation remains genuinely appropriate and important in this specific circumstance.

Board Alert Normal glucose, calcium, sodium, and cranial ultrasound do not exclude an inborn error of metabolism. The critical sample principle — timing collection to active decompensation — carries particular diagnostic importance.

Mock Exam 1 — Section B: Organ Systems | Universal Task 4: Management, Treatment and Prevention

Question 38

A 29-week gestation infant develops a significant, new heart murmur on day 3 of life along with bounding peripheral pulses and a widened pulse pressure.

Echocardiography confirms a haemodynamically significant patent ductus arteriosus with left atrial enlargement. Which of the following best reflects a currently accepted, evidence-based management consideration for this specific finding?

A. Every haemodynamically significant patent ductus arteriosus must be treated with immediate, surgical ligation regardless of any other, connected clinical consideration

B. Current management includes a range of approaches, from conservative, expectant management with close monitoring to pharmacologic closure or surgical ligation depending on this infant's own specific, connected clinical circumstance, reflecting genuinely current, ongoing evolution in this specific area's own evidence base

C. This finding carries no genuine, established relevance to this infant's own connected fluid or respiratory management of any kind

D. Pharmacologic closure represents the only medically acceptable approach in every specific circumstance, with no genuine role for observation

E. This finding requires no further, active clinical attention or connected management of any kind

Answer: B. **Current management ranges from conservative, expectant observation through pharmacologic closure to surgical ligation, depending on this infant's own specific, connected clinical circumstance — reflecting genuinely current, ongoing evolution in this evidence base.**

This vignette directly tests this book's own established cardiovascular content: management of a haemodynamically significant patent ductus arteriosus has genuinely, considerably evolved, with genuinely current evidence supporting a range of approaches rather than a single, uniform, reflexive intervention in every specific circumstance.

Correct, current practice requires actively weighing this infant's own specific, connected clinical circumstance — the genuine degree of haemodynamic significance, this infant's own respiratory status, and this same infant's own broader clinical trajectory together — rather than assuming immediate, surgical ligation represents the universally correct, single approach.

This reflects this book's own repeated theme that correctly, safely managing a genuinely important, connected cardiovascular finding requires individualised, evidence-based clinical judgment, honestly incorporating genuinely current, still-evolving evidence rather than a single, rigid, historical treatment algorithm.

Why the other options are wrong

A. A range of approaches, not universal, immediate surgical ligation, reflects genuinely current, evidence-based management.

C. This finding carries direct, established relevance to this infant's own broader, connected clinical management.

D. Conservative, expectant management retains a genuine, established role, not exclusively pharmacologic closure in every case.

E. This finding requires active, ongoing clinical attention and connected management, as detailed in the correct answer.

Board Alert Management of a haemodynamically significant PDA ranges from conservative observation through pharmacologic closure to surgical ligation, reflecting genuinely current, individualised, evidence-based clinical judgment.

Question 39

A term infant develops significant respiratory distress and is noted to have a scaphoid abdomen, absent breath sounds on the left, and bowel sounds audible within the left chest. Prenatal ultrasound had documented polyhydramnios. Genetic testing later confirms no chromosomal abnormality. Which of the following best reflects the single most important, connected prognostic determinant for this infant, beyond the diaphragmatic defect's own physical size alone?

A. This infant's specific chromosomal testing result represents the single most important, connected prognostic determinant in this specific circumstance

B. The genuine severity of pulmonary hypoplasia, directly connecting to foundational lung development physiology established throughout this book, frequently represents the single most genuinely important prognostic determinant for this infant, rather than the diaphragmatic defect's own physical size alone

C. Polyhydramnios carries no genuine, connected relevance to this infant's own eventual prognosis of any kind

D. This infant's own eventual prognosis is determined entirely, exclusively by this specific defect's own physical size alone

E. This infant's own respiratory presentation carries no genuine relevance to correctly determining prognosis

Answer: B. **The genuine severity of pulmonary hypoplasia, directly connecting to foundational lung development physiology, frequently represents the single most important prognostic determinant for this infant, rather than the diaphragmatic defect's own physical size alone.**

This vignette presents classic congenital diaphragmatic hernia, and this book's own repeated, cross-chapter theme directly applies: correctly, precisely grading the genuine severity of pulmonary hypoplasia, this specific, connected consequence directly extending the extensive lung development content established at length throughout this book's earlier volumes, carries direct, genuinely important relevance to correctly, completely evaluating this specific infant.

This specific, underlying lung development itself, rather than the diaphragmatic defect's own physical size alone, frequently represents the single most genuinely important determinant of this infant's own overall, eventual prognosis, reflecting this book's own repeated, cross-volume demonstration that a specific, foundational physiological principle directly explains why a given structural anomaly's own true clinical significance frequently extends well beyond its own simple, physical, anatomical description alone.

This does not mean chromosomal status carries no relevance whatsoever, but rather that in this specific infant, with confirmed, normal chromosomal testing, pulmonary hypoplasia severity specifically represents the single most important, connected prognostic consideration requiring active, careful evaluation.

Why the other options are wrong

A. In this specific infant, with normal chromosomal testing already confirmed, pulmonary hypoplasia severity represents the more directly relevant determinant.

C. Polyhydramnios carries direct, connected relevance to this infant's own presentation and evaluation.

D. Pulmonary hypoplasia severity, not defect size alone, frequently represents the single most important determinant.

E. This infant's own respiratory presentation carries direct, essential relevance to correctly determining prognosis.

Board Alert In congenital diaphragmatic hernia, the genuine severity of pulmonary hypoplasia, not the diaphragmatic defect's own physical size alone, frequently represents the single most important prognostic determinant.

Question 40

A 30-week gestation infant is 2 weeks old and has developed significant, progressive abdominal distension along with hypotonia and significant, delayed meconium passage. Total colonic aganglionosis is subsequently confirmed on rectal biopsy. Which of the following best reflects the correct, complete understanding of this specific diagnosis relative to a more typical, limited-segment presentation of this same condition?

- **A.** Total colonic aganglionosis carries an identical surgical approach and longer-term functional outcome to the more typical, limited-segment presentation
- **B.** This specific, more extensive variant, reflecting absent ganglion cells extending considerably further throughout the entire colon rather than a more limited, distal segment, generally carries a genuinely more complex surgical approach and correspondingly different, honest, longer-term functional outcome compared with the more typical, limited-segment presentation
- **C.** This specific variant reflects a genuinely more limited, rather than more extensive, degree of aganglionosis
- **D.** This specific diagnosis carries no genuine relationship to the foundational Hirschsprung disease mechanism
- **E.** This specific variant requires no genuine, specific distinction in surgical planning or family counselling

Answer: B. **Total colonic aganglionosis, reflecting absent ganglion cells extending throughout the entire colon, generally carries a genuinely more complex surgical approach and different, honest longer-term functional outcome compared with the more**

typical, limited-segment presentation.

This vignette directly tests this book's own extended surgical content: a total colonic aganglionosis variant represents a further, genuinely important, and genuinely more severe specific variant of Hirschsprung disease, reflecting genuine, absent ganglion cells extending considerably further, throughout the entire colon, rather than being confined to a more genuinely limited, distal segment.

This specific, more extensive variant generally carries a genuinely more complex, more challenging specific surgical approach and correspondingly, genuinely different longer-term functional outcome compared with the more typical, limited-segment presentation, directly informing both surgical planning and honest family counselling.

This reflects this book's own repeated theme that correctly, precisely characterising a given condition's own specific extent or severity directly informs the appropriate, individually tailored surgical approach and honest, longer-term prognostic counselling a given infant and family genuinely require.

Why the other options are wrong

A. This specific variant carries a genuinely more complex, not identical, surgical approach and outcome.

C. This reverses the correct relationship; this specific variant reflects a genuinely more extensive degree of aganglionosis.

D. This specific diagnosis has direct, mechanistic relevance to the foundational Hirschsprung disease mechanism.

E. This specific variant requires active, genuinely important distinction in both surgical planning and family counselling.

Board Alert Total colonic aganglionosis, a genuinely more severe Hirschsprung variant with absence extending throughout the entire colon, carries a genuinely more complex surgical approach and different, honest longer-term functional outcome.

Question 41

A genuinely current, specific research effort has directly examined transport-related mortality and morbidity specifically among paediatric patients supported on extracorporeal membrane oxygenation during genuine, active interhospital transfer. Which of the following best reflects the correct, honest interpretation of this specific research finding?

A. This specific finding should be treated as definitively, completely established, with no genuine, remaining limitation of any kind

B. This genuinely current research represents a genuinely important, though not yet completely, definitively established, contribution, drawn from a genuinely current, but still comparatively limited, single-centre and systematic review evidence base, warranting further, larger, multi-centre study

C. This specific research finding has no established basis in genuinely current, recently published literature of any kind

D. This specific research carries no genuine relevance to correctly, safely managing this specific combined process

E. A genuinely limited evidence base automatically, entirely invalidates this research's own genuine, practical clinical relevance

Answer: B. **This genuinely current research represents an important, though not yet definitively established, contribution, drawn from a comparatively limited evidence base, warranting further, larger, multi-centre study.**

This vignette directly tests this book's own honest, evidence-based approach to genuinely current transport and ECMO safety research: correctly, honestly acknowledging that this genuinely current research drew from a genuinely current, but still comparatively limited, single-centre and systematic review evidence base directly extends this book's own repeated theme of honest evidence treatment.

This means this genuinely current research represents a genuinely important, though not yet completely, definitively established, contribution to correctly understanding this specific, genuinely important clinical practice, warranting further, larger, multi-centre study, rather than being treated as though it carried false, complete certainty.

This reflects this book's own repeated, closing theme of honest, complete treatment of genuinely current evidence limitations, rather than presenting a genuinely important, current research finding as though its own, current conclusions were already, entirely, definitively settled.

Why the other options are wrong

A. Genuine, remaining limitation exists, as detailed in the correct answer, not definitive, complete establishment.

C. This specific research finding has direct, genuine basis in current, recently published literature.

D. This specific research carries direct, genuine relevance to this combined process, as detailed in the correct answer.

E. This limitation does not automatically invalidate practical relevance, as detailed in the correct answer.

Board Alert Genuinely current ECMO transport safety research represents an important, though not yet definitively established, contribution from a comparatively limited evidence base, warranting further, larger study.

Question 42

A term infant develops significant hypoglycaemia, microphallus, and midline facial anomalies including a single central incisor. Which of the following represents the most important, additional diagnostic consideration in this specific circumstance?

A. This presentation carries no genuine relationship to any specific, connected endocrine consideration of any kind

B. Active evaluation for congenital hypopituitarism should be pursued, given this infant's specific, connected combination of findings, since combined pituitary hormone deficiency can directly explain this exact, characteristic clinical pattern including significant, connected hypoglycaemia

C. This presentation should be managed exclusively as isolated, transient neonatal hypoglycaemia, without further, specific evaluation

D. Microphallus in this specific context carries no genuine, diagnostic significance of any kind

E. Midline facial anomalies carry no genuine, established relationship to any specific, underlying endocrine or structural consideration

Answer: B. Active evaluation for congenital hypopituitarism should be pursued, since combined pituitary hormone deficiency

directly explains this exact, characteristic combination of hypoglycaemia, microphallus, and midline facial anomalies.

This vignette presents the classic, connected combination for congenital hypopituitarism: significant hypoglycaemia reflecting combined growth hormone and cortisol deficiency, microphallus reflecting deficient gonadotropin stimulation during fetal development, and midline facial anomalies reflecting a connected, underlying disruption of midline brain and pituitary development together.

This connected reasoning — recognising that a single, underlying developmental disruption directly explains multiple, apparently distinct findings together — represents exactly the kind of mechanism-first, cross-system diagnostic reasoning this book has modelled throughout its own endocrine and genetics content.

Correctly, rapidly recognising this connected pattern directly supports urgent, active endocrine evaluation and appropriate hormone replacement, since untreated, combined pituitary hormone deficiency carries genuine, significant risk, particularly through unrecognised, significant hypoglycaemia and cortisol deficiency together.

Why the other options are wrong

A. This presentation carries a direct, well-established relationship to a specific, connected endocrine consideration.

C. This presentation warrants active, specific evaluation for a connected, underlying diagnosis, not management as isolated, transient hypoglycaemia.

D. This specific finding carries direct, diagnostic significance in this connected presentation, as detailed in the correct answer.

E. A direct, established relationship exists between these findings and this underlying, structural developmental consideration.

Board Alert Hypoglycaemia, microphallus, and midline facial anomalies together suggest congenital hypopituitarism, reflecting a connected, underlying disruption of midline brain and pituitary development.

Mock Exam 1 — Section B: Organ Systems | Universal Task 4: Management, Treatment and Prevention

Question 43

A 27-week gestation infant is 5 weeks old and has an ongoing, structured iron deficiency screening evaluation using reticulocyte haemoglobin content as part of a quality improvement initiative. Which of the following best reflects the connected, longer-term rationale for this specific screening effort?

A. This specific screening effort carries relevance exclusively to this infant's own immediate haematological status alone

B. This specific screening initiative carries genuine, connected relevance to neuroprotection, since iron carries genuine, established importance for normal, healthy neurodevelopment, directly connecting this specific quality improvement target to this infant's own broader, longer-term developmental outcome

C. Iron carries no genuine, established relationship to neurodevelopment of any kind

D. This specific screening effort has no genuine, connected relevance to this infant's own longer-term outcome of any kind

E. This specific quality improvement initiative carries no established basis in genuinely current literature of any kind

Answer: B. **This screening initiative carries genuine, connected relevance to neuroprotection, since iron carries genuine, established importance for normal, healthy neurodevelopment — directly connecting this quality improvement target to longer-term developmental outcome.**

This vignette directly tests this book's own genuinely current care systems and quality improvement content: iron deficiency screening, established as part of a genuinely important, structured quality improvement initiative, carries direct, genuine, connected relevance to neuroprotection.

This means this same, specific mineral carries genuine, established importance for normal, healthy neurodevelopment, directly connecting this earlier case study's own specific, quality improvement target to a genuinely important, foundational physiological principle established elsewhere throughout this book.

This reflects this book's own repeated theme that a specific quality improvement initiative's own genuine value frequently extends well beyond its own immediate, specific metric alone, to a further, genuinely important, connected physiological outcome — in this case, directly connecting a haematological screening effort to this infant's own longer-term, connected neurodevelopmental trajectory.

Why the other options are wrong

A. This screening carries genuine, connected relevance extending beyond immediate haematological status alone, as detailed in the correct answer.

C. A direct, established relationship exists between iron and neurodevelopment, as detailed in the correct answer.

D. This screening effort carries direct, genuine relevance to this infant's own longer-term outcome, as detailed in the correct answer.

E. This specific initiative has direct, genuine basis in genuinely current, published literature.

Board Alert Iron deficiency screening carries genuine, connected relevance to neuroprotection, since iron carries established importance for normal, healthy neurodevelopment — connecting a haematological target to longer-term outcome.

Question 44

A term infant born to a mother with confirmed, active genital herpes simplex virus infection at the time of vaginal delivery develops vesicular skin lesions on day 6 of life. Which of the following represents the most appropriate, immediate next step in this infant's evaluation and management?

A. No further evaluation is required, since isolated skin lesions in this context carry no genuine, connected significance

B. This presentation should prompt urgent evaluation for neonatal herpes simplex virus infection, including assessment for disease extent (skin, eye, and mouth alone versus disseminated or central nervous system involvement), with prompt initiation of intravenous acyclovir given this infection's own genuine potential for significant, rapid progression

C. This presentation should be managed exclusively with topical therapy alone, without any further, systemic evaluation or treatment

D. Maternal infection status carries no genuine relevance to correctly evaluating this specific infant's own presentation

E. This presentation should be observed for several additional days before any active, specific evaluation is pursued

Answer: B. This presentation should prompt urgent evaluation for neonatal herpes simplex virus infection, assessing disease

extent and promptly initiating intravenous acyclovir, given this infection's genuine potential for significant, rapid progression.

This vignette presents classic, high-risk neonatal herpes simplex virus infection, directly connecting to confirmed, active maternal genital infection at the time of vaginal delivery — a specific, well-established, elevated transmission risk scenario this book has established at length throughout its own infectious diseases content.

Correct, urgent evaluation directly requires assessing this infection's own specific extent, since neonatal herpes simplex virus infection can present across a genuinely important spectrum, from localised skin, eye, and mouth disease through to disseminated infection or central nervous system involvement, each carrying genuinely different, connected prognostic and treatment implications.

Prompt initiation of intravenous acyclovir represents the correct, urgent, established treatment, given this infection's own genuine, well-recognised potential for significant, rapid progression, meaning correctly, rapidly recognising this connected clinical pattern directly supports urgent, rather than delayed, evaluation and treatment.

Why the other options are wrong

A. This presentation carries genuine, significant connected significance, warranting active, urgent evaluation.

C. Systemic evaluation and treatment, not topical therapy alone, represents the correct, appropriate approach given this infection's potential severity.

D. Maternal infection status carries direct, essential relevance to correctly evaluating this infant's own presentation and risk.

E. This presentation warrants urgent, immediate evaluation, not observation over several additional days.

Board Alert Neonatal herpes simplex virus infection requires urgent evaluation of disease extent (skin/eye/mouth, disseminated, or CNS) and prompt intravenous acyclovir, given genuine potential for significant, rapid progression.

Mock Exam 1 — Section B: Organ Systems | Universal Task 4: Management, Treatment and Prevention

Question 45

A 26-week gestation infant is 4 weeks old and remains on continuous positive airway pressure. The clinical team is discussing sedation and analgesia for an upcoming, minor bedside procedure. Which of the following best reflects the correct, evidence-based approach to selecting and monitoring this specific medication?

A. Clinical impression alone represents an entirely sufficient, appropriate approach to guiding this specific medication decision, with no genuine value from any specific, validated scoring tool

B. Correctly, actively using a specific, validated pain and sedation scoring tool, together with active application of this infant's own genuinely distinctive developmental pharmacokinetic principles, represents the correct, structured approach, rather than relying on unstructured, purely subjective clinical judgment alone

C. This infant's own specific gestational age carries no genuine relevance to correctly selecting or dosing this specific medication

D. Every specific neonatal patient can be correctly, safely managed using an identical, standardised sedation regimen regardless of individual, developmental consideration

E. This specific procedure requires no genuine, active pain or sedation assessment of any kind

Answer: B. **Correctly using a validated pain and sedation scoring tool, together with this infant's own developmental pharmacokinetic principles, represents the correct, structured approach, not unstructured, purely subjective clinical judgment alone.**

This vignette directly tests this book's own established pharmacology content: correctly, actively using a specific, validated pain and sedation scoring tool provides a genuinely important, structured, and considerably more objective approach to guiding sedation and analgesia decisions than clinical impression alone.

This same, structured approach directly requires active application of this book's own extensively established developmental pharmacokinetic principles — this population's own genuinely distinctive drug handling, reduced hepatic blood flow, and receptor and enzyme ontogeny together — rather than assuming an identical, standardised regimen applies uniformly across every specific patient.

This reflects this book's own repeated theme that correctly, safely applying sedation and analgesia in this genuinely vulnerable population requires both structured, objective clinical assessment and active, individualised, developmentally aware pharmacological judgment together.

Why the other options are wrong

A. A specific, validated tool provides genuine, additional value, as detailed in the correct answer, not clinical impression alone.

C. This infant's own gestational age carries direct, essential relevance to correctly selecting and dosing this medication.

D. Individualised, developmental consideration is genuinely required, not an identical, standardised regimen for every patient.

E. Active pain and sedation assessment remains genuinely important for this specific procedure.

Board Alert Correctly managing procedural sedation requires both a validated pain and sedation scoring tool and active application of developmental pharmacokinetic principles — not clinical impression or a standardised regimen alone.

Question 46

A 25-week gestation infant develops significant, established necrotising enterocolitis with significant, otherwise unexplained metabolic acidosis. Which of the following best explains the connected, underlying mechanism most likely responsible for this specific acid-base finding?

A. This finding carries no genuine, connected relationship to this infant's own underlying necrotising enterocolitis of any kind

B. Significant bowel ischaemia directly produces lactate accumulation through anaerobic cellular metabolism, as inadequate tissue oxygen delivery forces affected cells to shift away from normal, aerobic metabolism, directly explaining this infant's own connected, significant metabolic acidosis and correspondingly elevated anion gap

C. This specific finding reflects a primary respiratory, rather than metabolic, disturbance entirely unrelated to this infant's own bowel pathology

D. Lactate accumulation carries no genuine, mechanistic relationship to significant bowel ischaemia of any kind

E. This specific acid-base finding requires no further, active clinical correlation with this infant's own underlying condition

Answer: B. Significant bowel ischaemia directly produces lactate accumulation through anaerobic metabolism, as inadequate tissue oxygen delivery forces cells away from aerobic metabolism, directly explaining this infant's connected, significant metabolic acidosis and elevated anion gap.

This vignette directly tests this book's own connected acid-base and surgical content: significant, established necrotising enterocolitis represents a further, specific, genuinely important cause of significant metabolic acidosis, reflecting the combination of significant bowel ischaemia directly producing lactate accumulation.

This same mechanism directly connects to this book's own foundational content regarding elevated anion gap: significant, prolonged hypoperfusion directly produces significant metabolic acidosis through anaerobic cellular metabolism, as inadequate tissue oxygen delivery forces cells to genuinely shift away from normal, considerably more efficient aerobic metabolism.

This reflects this book's own repeated theme that correctly, actively recognising significant, otherwise unexplained metabolic acidosis in a given infant should specifically, actively prompt consideration of this specific, genuinely serious gastrointestinal condition among the broader, connected differential diagnosis.

Why the other options are wrong

A. A direct, well-established, mechanistic relationship exists between these two findings, as detailed in the correct answer.

C. This finding reflects a primary metabolic, not respiratory, disturbance, directly connected to this infant's own bowel pathology.

D. A direct, mechanistic relationship exists between bowel ischaemia and lactate accumulation, as detailed in the correct answer.

E. Active, ongoing clinical correlation with this infant's own underlying condition remains genuinely important.

Board Alert Significant bowel ischaemia in necrotising enterocolitis directly produces lactate accumulation through anaerobic metabolism, explaining connected, significant metabolic acidosis and an elevated anion gap.

Question 47

A 28-week gestation infant is being evaluated for possible retinopathy of prematurity treatment. The family asks about this infant's own longer-term visual prognosis. Which of the following best reflects the correct, honest, and complete response to this specific family question?

A. This infant's own longer-term visual outcome can be predicted with entirely complete, absolute certainty at this specific point in this infant's own clinical course

B. Honest, complete counselling requires acknowledging genuine, remaining uncertainty regarding this infant's own specific, eventual visual outcome, while also actively committing to the same structured, serial ophthalmologic surveillance this book has established as essential for correctly, safely guiding treatment decisions and monitoring this same, genuine trajectory over time

C. This specific family question deserves no genuine, substantive response of any kind

D. This infant's own current retinopathy of prematurity findings carry no genuine relevance to this infant's own longer-term visual prognosis

E. Structured, serial ophthalmologic surveillance carries no genuine relevance to correctly addressing this specific family question

Answer: B. **Honest, complete counselling requires acknowledging genuine, remaining uncertainty regarding eventual visual outcome, while committing to the same structured, serial surveillance this book establishes as essential for guiding treatment decisions over time.**

This vignette directly tests this book's own repeated, honest communication principle applied to a genuinely important, common family question: correctly, compassionately responding requires honestly acknowledging genuine, remaining uncertainty regarding this infant's own specific, eventual visual outcome, rather than offering false, absolute certainty.

This same, honest response directly connects to this book's own established retinopathy of prematurity content: structured, serial ophthalmologic examinations must continue on an individualised schedule, since this condition can genuinely progress, this same, ongoing surveillance directly informing the correct, timely treatment decision should progression genuinely occur.

This reflects this book's own repeated theme that honest, complete communication with a family requires actively acknowledging genuine uncertainty while still providing this same family with a clear, concrete, and genuinely reassuring plan for ongoing, structured, and connected clinical attention.

Why the other options are wrong

A. Genuine, remaining uncertainty exists at this stage, as detailed in the correct answer, not entirely complete, absolute certainty.

C. This specific family question deserves a genuine, substantive, honest response, as detailed in the correct answer.

D. This infant's own current findings carry direct, genuine relevance to this infant's own longer-term prognosis.

E. This surveillance carries direct, genuine relevance to addressing this specific family question, as detailed in the correct answer.

Board Alert Honest counselling on retinopathy of prematurity prognosis acknowledges genuine, remaining uncertainty while committing to structured, serial surveillance to guide treatment decisions over time.

Question 48

A genuinely current, specific study directly compares a new screening intervention against usual care in a cohort of preterm infants, reporting the intervention's own sensitivity and specificity for detecting a specific, important condition. Which of the following statements about correctly, completely interpreting this specific study's own reported statistics is most accurate?

A. Sensitivity and specificity alone provide an entirely complete picture of this test's own genuine, clinical usefulness in every specific circumstance

B. Sensitivity and specificity, while genuinely important and independent of this condition's own prevalence, should be complemented by positive and negative predictive value, which genuinely, directly depend on this same condition's own actual, underlying prevalence within the specific population genuinely being screened

C. Positive and negative predictive value carry no genuine, meaningful relationship to a given condition's own prevalence of any kind

D. This specific distinction carries no genuine, meaningful relevance to correctly, completely interpreting this study's own reported findings

E. Sensitivity and specificity genuinely, directly depend on this condition's own prevalence, identically to positive and negative predictive value

Answer: B. **Sensitivity and specificity, genuinely independent of prevalence, should be complemented by positive and negative predictive value, which genuinely, directly depend on this condition's own actual, underlying prevalence within the specific population being screened.**

This vignette directly tests this book's own foundational diagnostic test statistics content: sensitivity, the genuine proportion of truly affected individuals correctly identified as positive, and specificity, the genuine proportion of truly unaffected individuals correctly identified as negative, together characterise a given test's own overall, genuine performance.

Positive predictive value and negative predictive value represent two further, genuinely distinct properties: correctly, precisely interpreting either of these two properties directly depends on the specific condition's own actual, underlying prevalence, unlike sensitivity and specificity, which genuinely remain independent of this same prevalence.

This means correctly, completely evaluating this specific screening intervention requires actively considering multiple, genuinely distinct statistical properties together, each carrying its own, genuinely different practical implication for this specific population's own actual, underlying disease prevalence.

Why the other options are wrong

A. These two properties alone provide an incomplete picture; predictive values, dependent on prevalence, are also required.

C. A direct, essential relationship exists between predictive value and prevalence, as detailed in the correct answer.

D. This specific distinction carries direct, essential relevance to completely interpreting this study, as detailed in the correct answer.

E. This reverses the correct relationship; sensitivity and specificity remain independent of prevalence, unlike predictive values.

Board Alert Sensitivity and specificity are independent of prevalence. Positive and negative predictive value genuinely depend on the specific population's own actual, underlying disease prevalence.

Question 49

A term infant develops significant, progressive jaundice with acholic stools by 3 weeks of life. Direct bilirubin comprises 45 per cent of the total, and abdominal ultrasound shows an absent gallbladder. Which of the following represents the most appropriate, immediate next step?

A. Reassurance and continued observation alone, since this presentation likely reflects a self-limited, physiologic process requiring no further, urgent evaluation

B. Urgent evaluation for biliary atresia, including consideration of hepatobiliary scintigraphy or direct surgical exploration, given this infant's specific combination of findings and this condition's own genuine, time-sensitive surgical treatment window

C. This presentation should be managed exclusively with phototherapy alone, without further, specific diagnostic evaluation

D. Acholic stools carry no genuine, diagnostic significance in this specific clinical context

E. This presentation should be observed for several additional weeks before any active, specific evaluation is pursued

Answer: B. **This presentation warrants urgent evaluation for biliary atresia, given this specific combination of findings and this condition's own genuine, time-sensitive surgical treatment window — not reassurance, phototherapy, or delayed observation.**

This vignette presents classic biliary atresia: progressive, direct hyperbilirubinaemia, acholic stools reflecting genuine biliary obstruction, and an absent or abnormal gallbladder on ultrasound together, occurring at an age directly relevant to this condition's own genuine, time-sensitive treatment window.

This presentation directly requires urgent, rather than delayed, evaluation, since biliary atresia's own genuine surgical treatment, the Kasai portoenterostomy, carries genuinely, considerably better outcomes when performed before approximately 8 weeks of age, making prompt recognition and evaluation directly, genuinely time-sensitive.

This reflects this book's own repeated theme that correctly, rapidly recognising a specific, connected clinical pattern — direct hyperbilirubinaemia with acholic stools specifically — directly changes the appropriate, immediate management approach, given this specific presentation's own genuine surgical urgency.

Why the other options are wrong

A. This presentation is genuinely concerning for a time-sensitive surgical condition, not a self-limited, physiologic process.

C. Phototherapy alone is not appropriate for a predominantly direct hyperbilirubinaemia; urgent, specific evaluation is required.

D. This specific finding carries direct, significant diagnostic significance in this specific clinical context.

E. This presentation warrants urgent, immediate evaluation, given this condition's own genuine, time-sensitive treatment window.

Board Alert Biliary atresia: progressive direct hyperbilirubinaemia, acholic stools, absent gallbladder. Requires urgent evaluation, given the Kasai portoenterostomy's genuinely better outcomes when performed before approximately 8 weeks of age.

Question 50

A genuinely current, specific randomised controlled trial enrolling preterm twins reports a significant benefit for a new intervention, with no explicit discussion of how this same trial accounted for the genuine, correlated relationship between co-enrolled twin pairs. Which of the following best reflects the correct, critical appraisal this specific finding requires?

A. This specific finding should be accepted entirely, uncritically, given its own reported statistical significance alone

B. This trial's own enrolment of twins requires active, critical scrutiny, since twins genuinely, statistically share a correlated relationship, including shared genetic and shared intrauterine environment, rather than representing genuinely, statistically independent observations, meaning correctly, appropriately analysing this trial's own data requires actively accounting for this same, genuine non-independence

C. Twins genuinely represent entirely, statistically independent observations, with no genuine, correlated relationship of any kind

D. This specific methodological consideration carries no genuine relevance to correctly, critically appraising this specific trial

E. This trial's own enrolment of twins carries no genuine, meaningful relevance to correctly analysing this trial's own actual data

Answer: B. This trial's own enrolment of twins requires active, critical scrutiny, since twins genuinely share a correlated relationship rather than representing statistically independent observations, requiring active accounting for this non-independence.

This vignette directly tests this book's own genuinely current methodological content: correctly accounting for multiple births within perinatal and neonatal clinical trials represents a genuinely important, specific challenge, since twins or triplets genuinely, statistically share a genuine, correlated relationship, including shared genetic and shared intrauterine environment.

This means correctly, appropriately analysing this same trial's own data requires actively accounting for this same, genuine, non-independence, rather than treating every specific infant as an entirely separate, independent data point — a genuinely current, specific methodological challenge this book has established as directly connecting to twin physiology content established at length elsewhere.

This reflects this book's own repeated, closing theme that correctly, rigorously analysing genuinely current research requires active attention to specific, sometimes subtle methodological detail genuinely specific to this particular, unique population, rather than uncritical acceptance of a single, favourable, reported result.

Why the other options are wrong

A. Uncritical acceptance is not warranted; active, critical scrutiny of this specific methodological consideration is required.

C. Twins genuinely share a correlated, not entirely independent, relationship, as detailed in the correct answer.

D. This specific consideration carries direct, essential relevance to critical appraisal, as detailed in the correct answer.

E. This enrolment carries direct, essential relevance to correctly analysing this trial's own data, as detailed in the correct answer.

Board Alert Twins or triplets genuinely share a correlated relationship rather than representing statistically independent observations, requiring active, critical scrutiny of how a given trial accounted for this non-independence.

Question 51

A term infant with confirmed, severe meconium aspiration syndrome and secondary persistent pulmonary hypertension, genuinely failing maximal conventional therapy, is being evaluated for extracorporeal membrane oxygenation. Which of the following configurations is generally preferred given this infant's predominantly respiratory pathology, and why?

A. Venoarterial configuration, since this configuration provides support for cardiac function alone, without any genuine, direct respiratory benefit

B. Venovenous configuration, since this configuration supports genuinely reversible respiratory failure specifically, without providing direct haemodynamic support, making it generally appropriate when an infant's underlying pathology is genuinely, predominantly respiratory rather than additionally, significantly cardiac

C. Neither configuration carries any genuine, meaningful distinction relevant to this specific clinical decision

D. Configuration selection carries no genuine relationship to whether a given infant's pathology is predominantly respiratory or cardiac

E. Venoarterial configuration is always, universally preferred regardless of an infant's own specific, underlying pathology

Answer: B. **Venovenous configuration is generally preferred here, since it supports genuinely reversible respiratory failure without providing direct haemodynamic support, appropriate for this infant's predominantly respiratory pathology.**

This vignette directly tests this book's own foundational ECMO content: venovenous extracorporeal membrane oxygenation, in which blood is withdrawn from and returned to the venous circulation alone, supports genuinely reversible respiratory failure specifically, without providing any genuine, direct haemodynamic support.

Venoarterial configuration, by contrast, provides genuine, direct support for both respiratory and cardiac function together, generally reserved for circumstances involving genuine, significant cardiac compromise alongside respiratory failure — a distinction genuinely relevant here, since this infant's pathology, while producing secondary pulmonary hypertension, remains predominantly, primarily respiratory in origin.

This reflects this book's own repeated theme that this single, foundational configuration distinction directly explains the entire, subsequent framework for correctly, appropriately selecting a given infant's own specific ECMO approach based on this infant's own actual, underlying pathology.

Why the other options are wrong

A. This reverses the correct relationship; venoarterial configuration provides combined support, not cardiac support alone without respiratory benefit.

C. A genuinely important, meaningful distinction exists between these two configurations, as detailed in the correct answer.

D. A direct, essential relationship exists between pathology type and configuration selection, as detailed in the correct answer.

E. Venovenous configuration is generally preferred for predominantly respiratory pathology, not venoarterial configuration universally.

Board Alert Venovenous ECMO supports genuinely reversible respiratory failure alone, appropriate for predominantly respiratory pathology. Venoarterial ECMO provides combined respiratory and cardiac support.

Question 52

A family whose infant has genuinely, actively been redirected toward comfort-focused care asks the clinical team whether they may have genuine, private time together before this infant's own anticipated death. Which of the following best reflects the correct, compassionate response to this specific request?

A. This request should be declined, since private family time carries no genuine, meaningful relevance to compassionate end-of-life care

B. This request should genuinely, actively be honoured whenever genuinely, practically possible, since correctly, compassionately supporting this family requires actively creating this same, genuine space, rather than this profound, final transition occurring within a genuinely impersonal, clinically dominated environment alone

C. This request carries no genuine relevance to this book's own established, family-centred communication principle

D. This family's own specific request should be deferred indefinitely without any genuine, active response

E. Clinical intervention alone should genuinely, entirely define this infant's own remaining, brief life

Answer: B. This request should genuinely be honoured whenever practically possible, since compassionately supporting this family requires creating this genuine space, rather than this final transition occurring within a purely clinical environment alone.

This vignette directly tests this book's own established ethics and palliative care content: correctly, compassionately allowing a family genuine, private time with this infant, whenever genuinely, practically possible, represents a genuinely important, specific consideration throughout redirection of care.

This same, genuine consideration directly extends this book's own honest, family-centred communication principle established repeatedly throughout, meaning correctly, compassionately supporting this family requires actively, deliberately creating this same, genuine space for connection.

This reflects this book's own repeated theme that this entire, genuinely sensitive field requires attention to the deeply human, as well as the clinical, dimension of a family's own genuine experience throughout every stage of this same, connected journey, including this infant's own final, remaining time.

Why the other options are wrong

A. This specific request carries direct, genuine relevance to compassionate end-of-life care, as detailed in the correct answer.

C. This request has direct, essential relevance to this book's own family-centred communication principle.

D. This request deserves an active, genuine, and generally affirming response, not indefinite deferral.

E. Genuine, further space for meaningful connection exists, as detailed in the correct answer, not exclusive clinical definition.

Board Alert Correctly, compassionately honouring a family's request for private time during redirection of care represents a genuinely important consideration, whenever practically possible.

Mock Exam 1 — Section C: Application | Universal Task 1: Core Science

Question 53

A specific, genuinely current guideline directly addresses routine neuromonitoring in the neonatal and paediatric patient supported on extracorporeal membrane oxygenation. Which of the following best explains the specific rationale underlying this genuinely current guideline?

A. This specific guideline reflects genuinely arbitrary, rather than evidence-based, professional preference

B. This genuinely current guideline directly reflects active, professional recognition of this technology's own genuine, connected neurological risk, meaning correctly, safely managing an infant receiving this technology requires active, structured neuromonitoring throughout support, rather than reactive evaluation only once overt, clinically apparent neurological injury has already occurred

C. This technology carries no genuine, connected neurological risk of any kind, making this specific guideline unnecessary

D. Reactive evaluation following overt, clinically apparent injury represents the genuinely preferred approach to neurological monitoring in this population

E. This specific guideline has no relationship to this technology's own genuine, connected risk profile of any kind

Answer: B. **This genuinely current guideline reflects active, professional recognition of ECMO's genuine, connected neurological risk, requiring active, structured neuromonitoring throughout support rather than reactive evaluation after overt injury has already occurred.**

This vignette directly tests this book's own genuinely current transport and ECMO content: this genuinely current guideline directly reflects active, professional recognition of this same technology's own genuine, connected neurological risk, itself directly relevant to significant intraventricular haemorrhage and hypoxic-ischaemic encephalopathy content established at length throughout this book's earlier volumes.

This means correctly, safely managing an infant receiving this chapter's own central technology requires active, structured neuromonitoring throughout the entire duration of support, rather than reactive evaluation only once overt, clinically apparent neurological injury has already, genuinely occurred.

This reflects this book's own repeated theme that correctly, safely applying a genuinely powerful clinical technology requires active, proactive clinical vigilance extending well beyond this technology's own immediate, direct physiological support alone.

Why the other options are wrong

A. This specific guideline has direct, genuine, evidence-based rationale, as detailed in the correct answer, not arbitrary preference.

C. A genuine, connected neurological risk exists, as detailed in the correct answer, directly justifying this specific guideline.

D. Active, structured monitoring, not reactive evaluation, represents the genuinely preferred, current approach.

E. This specific guideline has direct, essential relevance to this technology's own genuine, connected risk profile.

Board Alert Genuinely current ECMO neuromonitoring guidelines reflect active, professional recognition of this technology's genuine, connected neurological risk, requiring proactive, structured monitoring rather than reactive evaluation.

Question 54

A Level II neonatal intensive care unit identifies a genuinely important opportunity to improve its own outbreak preparedness following a recent, significant bacterial outbreak. Which of the following combined elements would most directly reflect the genuinely current, evidence-based framework this book establishes for structured outbreak management?

A. A single, isolated intervention alone, without any further, structured or combined component

B. A structured, Plan-Do-Study-Act-based framework combining early-warning triggers, multidisciplinary task-force activation, environmental decontamination protocols, and real-time auditing with structured feedback together

C. This specific unit's own genuine staffing status carries no genuine relevance to correctly implementing this specific framework

D. Reactive, rather than proactive, response alone represents the genuinely preferred, evidence-based approach to outbreak management

E. This specific framework carries no established basis in genuinely current, recently published quality improvement literature

Answer: B. A structured, PDSA-based framework combining early-warning triggers, multidisciplinary task-force activation, environmental decontamination, and real-time auditing together most directly reflects the genuinely current, evidence-based outbreak management framework this book establishes.

This vignette directly tests this book's own genuinely current care systems and quality improvement content: a genuinely current quality improvement evaluation directly found that a structured, Plan-Do-Study-Act-based framework, incorporating early-warning triggers and multidisciplinary task-force activation, directly, measurably improved outbreak containment compared with an earlier, more reactive approach.

This same, comprehensive framework directly incorporates further, genuinely important components established throughout this book's own broader content: environmental decontamination protocols directly complementing these earlier components, and real-time auditing with structured feedback directly reinforcing the foundational Plan-Do-Study-Act cycle's own "Study" phase, applied continuously throughout an active, ongoing circumstance.

This reflects this book's own repeated theme that a genuinely effective quality improvement framework frequently combines multiple, genuinely distinct, complementary structural components together, rather than any single, isolated measure considered on its own.

Why the other options are wrong

A. A single, isolated intervention does not reflect the genuinely comprehensive, combined framework this book establishes.

C. This unit's own staffing status carries genuine, practical relevance to implementing this framework effectively.

D. Proactive, structured response, not reactive response alone, represents the genuinely preferred, evidence-based approach.

E. This specific framework has direct, genuine basis in genuinely current, published quality improvement literature.

Board Alert A comprehensive, structured outbreak management framework combines early-warning triggers, multidisciplinary task-force activation, environmental decontamination, and real-time auditing together, within a Plan-Do-Study-Act structure.

Question 55

A genuinely current, specific systematic review evidence base has directly examined extracorporeal membrane oxygenation's own application to significant maternal acute respiratory distress syndrome during pregnancy. Which of the following best reflects this specific, genuinely current finding?

A. This technology has no established, specific relationship to significant maternal acute respiratory distress syndrome during pregnancy of any kind

B. This genuinely current systematic review found maternal survival genuinely ranging from 33 to 100 per cent across the specific studies examined, with larger, more recent series specifically reporting survival exceeding 80 per cent, directly extending this technology's own genuinely important relevance beyond the neonate alone

C. This specific systematic review found maternal survival to be uniformly, consistently below 50 per cent across every specific study examined

D. This specific research finding has no established basis in genuinely current, recently published systematic review evidence of any kind

E. This specific connection has no relationship to content established at length throughout this book's own maternal-fetal medicine content

Answer: B. **This genuinely current systematic review found maternal survival ranging from 33 to 100 per cent, with larger, more recent series reporting survival exceeding 80 per cent — directly extending this technology's genuinely important relevance beyond the neonate alone.**

This vignette directly tests this book's own genuinely fascinating, current cross-volume connection: genuinely current systematic review evidence, incorporating literature searched through May 2025, has directly examined this same technology's own application to significant maternal acute respiratory distress syndrome during pregnancy.

This specific systematic review found maternal survival genuinely ranging from 33 to 100 per cent across the specific studies examined, with larger, more recent series specifically reporting survival exceeding 80 per cent, reinforcing this book's repeated, cross-volume demonstration that a specific technology established at length in one chapter carries direct, genuinely unexpected relevance extending well beyond the neonate alone.

This directly connects to this book's own extensive maternal-fetal medicine content established throughout its earlier volume, illustrating this book's repeated theme that this same technology's own genuine, connected relevance extends to the maternal patient as well as this infant this book has otherwise, primarily addressed.

Why the other options are wrong

A. A direct, well-established relationship exists, as detailed in the correct answer, not an absence of relationship.

C. This specific review found survival genuinely ranging widely, with more recent series exceeding 80 per cent, not uniformly below 50 per cent.

D. This specific research finding has direct, genuine basis in current, recently published systematic review evidence.

E. This specific connection has direct, mechanistic relevance to content established at length throughout this book.

Board Alert A genuinely current systematic review of ECMO for maternal ARDS during pregnancy found maternal survival ranging from 33 to 100 per cent, with more recent series exceeding 80 per cent.

Question 56

A genuinely current, specific randomised controlled trial and a specific, case-control study each separately examine the same, specific perinatal exposure and outcome. Which of the following best explains why these two, genuinely distinct study designs might be expected to produce genuinely different specific measures of association?

A. A randomised controlled trial and a case-control study genuinely, always produce an identical, single specific measure of association

B. A randomised controlled trial, and the cohort design it shares its underlying structure with, directly produces relative risk, while a case-control study typically produces an odds ratio instead, reflecting these two designs' own genuinely different, underlying data structure and analytic approach

C. This specific distinction carries no genuine, meaningful relevance to correctly interpreting these two, genuinely different specific studies

D. A case-control study genuinely, typically produces relative risk, reversing the correct relationship established in this specific context

E. The specific study design used carries no genuine relationship to which specific measure of association a given study actually produces

Answer: B. A randomised controlled trial, sharing its underlying structure with a cohort design, directly produces relative risk, while a case-control study typically produces an odds ratio, reflecting these two designs' own genuinely different data structure.

This vignette directly tests this book's own foundational biostatistics content: relative risk, the genuine ratio of a given outcome's own actual incidence in an exposed group compared with an unexposed group, is directly calculated within a cohort study or randomised trial.

An odds ratio, the genuine ratio of a given outcome's own actual odds between these same two comparison groups, is typically, genuinely calculated within a case-control study instead, this second measure reflecting this specific design's own genuinely different, backward-looking data structure, beginning with already-identified cases rather than a forward-followed, defined cohort.

This reflects this book's own repeated theme that correctly, precisely understanding this specific distinction directly informs which specific measure a given study design actually, appropriately produces, and correctly, critically interpreting a given comparative finding requires actively considering this same, underlying study design.

Why the other options are wrong

A. These two designs genuinely produce genuinely different, specific measures, not an identical, single measure.

C. This specific distinction carries direct, essential relevance to correctly interpreting these two studies, as detailed in the correct answer.

D. This reverses the correct relationship; a case-control study typically produces an odds ratio, not relative risk.

E. A direct, essential relationship exists between design and measure, as detailed in the correct answer.

Board Alert A cohort study or randomised trial directly produces relative risk. A case-control study typically produces an odds ratio, reflecting these two designs' own genuinely different underlying data structure.

Question 57

A genuinely current survey has directly documented a significant nursing staff shortage occurring alongside a simultaneous, significant increase in board-certified neonatologist numbers, together with a genuinely improving ratio of ventilators to intensive care beds. Which of the following best reflects the correct, complete interpretation of these combined, connected findings?

A. Every specific systems-level indicator genuinely, always moves in an identical, proportional direction together, with no genuine, meaningful divergence of any kind possible

B. Correctly, honestly understanding this system's own broader status requires actively recognising that equipment capacity, physician staffing, and nursing staffing can genuinely, independently diverge, rather than assuming these genuinely distinct systems-level considerations always move together in an identical, connected direction

C. This combination of findings carries no genuine, meaningful relevance to correctly understanding this system's own overall status

D. Nursing staffing carries no genuine, independent relevance distinct from physician staffing or equipment capacity

E. This specific combination of findings has no established basis in genuinely current, published survey evidence of any kind

Answer: B. **Correctly understanding this system's status requires recognising that equipment capacity, physician staffing, and nursing staffing can genuinely, independently diverge, rather than assuming these distinct considerations always move together.**

This vignette directly tests this book's own genuinely current, honest care systems content: genuinely current, specific survey evidence has directly documented a significant nursing staff shortage occurring despite a simultaneous, significant increase in board-certified neonatologist numbers over the same, extended study period.

This same survey evidence has separately documented a significantly improving ratio of ventilators to intensive care beds occurring alongside this same nursing shortage, meaning correctly, honestly understanding this system's own broader status requires actively recognising that equipment capacity and staffing capacity can genuinely, independently diverge.

This reflects this book's own repeated theme that correctly, safely operating a regionalized system of care requires active, honest attention to multiple, genuinely distinct, and sometimes divergent, systems-level dimensions together, rather than physician numbers or equipment metrics alone providing a genuinely complete picture.

Why the other options are wrong

A. Genuine, meaningful divergence is genuinely possible, as detailed in the correct answer, not identical, proportional movement always.

C. This combination carries direct, genuine relevance to understanding this system's own overall status.

D. Nursing staffing carries genuine, independent relevance distinct from these other considerations, as detailed in the correct answer.

E. This specific combination has direct, genuine basis in current, published survey evidence.

Board Alert Equipment capacity, physician staffing, and nursing staffing can genuinely, independently diverge — a genuinely current survey documented a significant nursing shortage occurring alongside both increased neonatologist numbers and an improving ventilator-to-bed ratio.

Question 58

A family caring for an infant genuinely receiving perinatal palliative care asks the clinical team about neonatal organ donation as a specific option. Which of the following best reflects the correct, compassionate approach to this specific conversation?

A. This specific option should never, under any circumstance, be discussed with any family of any kind

B. This specific consideration requires the same, careful, honest, and transparent approach this book establishes throughout as its own foundational, central approach, meaning correctly, compassionately discussing this specific, genuinely sensitive option with this family requires the same, careful attention to this family's own genuine values this book has emphasised throughout its entire content

C. This specific consideration should be approached with a genuinely different, less careful communication standard than the rest of this book's own established content

D. This family's own genuine interest in this specific option carries no genuine relevance to correctly, compassionately responding to this specific question

E. This specific consideration carries no genuine, established relationship to shared decision-making of any kind

Answer: B. This specific consideration requires the same careful, honest, and transparent approach this book establishes throughout as its foundational approach, with the same careful attention to this family's own genuine values.

This vignette directly tests this book's own established ethics content: neonatal organ donation represents a specific, genuinely important ethical consideration directly extending the shared decision-making content established throughout this book, this specific consideration genuinely requiring the same, careful, honest, and transparent approach.

This means correctly, compassionately discussing this specific, genuinely sensitive option with this family requires the same, careful attention to this family's own genuine values this book has emphasised throughout its own entire span, rather than this specific topic being treated as somehow separate or exempt from this book's own foundational communication standard.

This reflects this book's own repeated theme that its own foundational, shared decision-making approach applies with equal, genuine care to every specific, sensitive topic this book addresses, rather than this same, foundational approach being reserved for only certain, specific circumstances.

Why the other options are wrong

A. This specific option can genuinely, appropriately be discussed with an interested family, not universally excluded.

C. This same, careful communication standard applies consistently, not a genuinely different, less careful standard.

D. This family's own genuine interest carries direct, essential relevance to this conversation, as detailed in the correct answer.

E. This specific consideration has direct, essential relevance to shared decision-making, as detailed in the correct answer.

Board Alert Neonatal organ donation, when raised by a family, requires the same careful, honest, transparent, shared decision-making approach this book establishes as foundational to every sensitive topic it addresses.

Question 59

A 24-week gestation infant, genuinely struggling within a Level II facility experiencing significant nursing shortage, requires transfer to a Level III facility for a genuinely higher level of subspecialty care. Which of the following best reflects the correct, complete approach to this specific transfer?

A. This transfer requires no genuine, structured pre-transport checklist, relying entirely on individual, unstructured clinical judgment alone

B. This transfer requires correctly, safely securing this infant's own airway and vascular access before movement actually begins, actively extending this book's own thermal management principles into this genuinely challenging, mobile environment, and following a coordinated, structured pre-transport checklist directly extending this book's repeated, coordinated care principle

C. This infant's own specific facility level carries no genuine relevance to correctly planning this specific transfer

D. Thermal management principles carry no genuine relevance to this specific, mobile transport environment

E. This specific transfer can be correctly, safely managed without any genuine, structured preparation of any kind

Answer: B. **This transfer requires securing airway and vascular access before movement begins, actively extending thermal management principles into this mobile environment, and following a coordinated, structured pre-transport checklist.**

This vignette directly tests this book's own established transport content: correctly, safely securing the airway and stable vascular access before genuine, active transport actually begins is essential, since correction becomes considerably more difficult once movement has already begun.

This same transport directly requires actively, proactively extending this book's own extensively established thermal management principles into this specific, genuinely challenging mobile environment, since this same environment carries its own, genuine, elevated risk of significant heat loss.

Correctly, safely preparing this infant for genuine, active transport directly requires a coordinated, structured pre-transport checklist, directly extending the structured team communication and coordinated care principles established repeatedly throughout this entire book, rather than an unstructured, individually variable approach.

Why the other options are wrong

A. A genuine, structured checklist is required, as detailed in the correct answer, not individual judgment alone without structure.

C. This infant's own facility level carries direct, genuine relevance to planning this transfer, as detailed in the correct answer.

D. These principles carry direct, particular importance in this specific, mobile environment, as detailed in the correct answer.

E. Genuine, structured preparation is required for this specific transfer, as detailed in the correct answer.

Board Alert Safe interhospital transfer requires securing airway and vascular access before movement begins, extending thermal management principles into the mobile environment, and following a coordinated, structured pre-transport checklist.

Question 60

This is the final question of Mock Exam 1. A 24-week gestation infant with confirmed, severe persistent pulmonary hypertension is being evaluated for extracorporeal membrane oxygenation at a referring, Level II facility. This infant's family is present and asking detailed questions about this proposed intervention's genuine risk, while the clinical team simultaneously debates whether genuinely current, portable ECMO technology should be used to cannulate this infant at this same referring facility before transport. Which of the following best reflects the complete, correct, and coordinated approach to this entire, connected circumstance?

A. This infant should genuinely, always be transported to a specialised facility first, with ECMO considered only after arrival, and this family's questions should genuinely be deferred until after this same intervention has already begun

B. Recognise that this infant's own extremely preterm status represents a specific, relative contraindication given compounded bleeding vulnerability, requiring active risk-benefit weighing against this technology's own genuine, potential benefit for this confirmed, severe condition; recognise that genuinely current, portable technology may enable safe, on-site cannulation before transport, requiring the specialised, coordinated mobile ECMO team this circumstance demands; recognise that correctly, safely applying this technology requires the coordinated, multidisciplinary team and active neuromonitoring this book establishes throughout; and recognise that this family's detailed questions deserve the same honest, calibrated, shared decision-making communication this book has modelled throughout its entire span

C. This infant's own extremely preterm status carries no genuine relevance to correctly determining candidacy for this technology

D. This family's own detailed questions should genuinely, entirely be deferred until this specific procedure has already, fully concluded

E. This genuinely complex, combined circumstance can be correctly, safely managed by a single specialist acting entirely independently, without genuine, coordinated involvement of any kind

Answer: B. **Every principle across this entire exam converges here: the connected relative contraindication requiring careful weighing, the genuinely current technology potentially enabling on-site cannulation, the coordinated team and active neuromonitoring this technology requires, and the honest, shared decision-making communication this family deserves throughout.**

This truly final question of Mock Exam 1 is deliberately constructed to require synthesis across essentially every domain this exam has addressed — foundations, organ systems, and application together — exactly as the certifying examination itself, and real clinical practice, ultimately demand.

This infant's own extremely preterm status directly raises the specific, relative contraindication established throughout this book's ECMO content, given this technology's own required anticoagulation compounding this population's already elevated, established bleeding vulnerability, requiring active, careful weighing of this connected risk against this technology's own genuine, potential benefit for this infant's own confirmed, severe condition.

Correctly, safely applying this technology, should candidacy genuinely be confirmed, requires the same coordinated, multidisciplinary team and connected neuromonitoring established throughout this book, while this family's own detailed, difficult questions deserve the same honest, calibrated, shared decision-making communication this entire book has modelled throughout its complete, three-volume span — closing this exam on precisely the standard of connected, compassionate synthesis this entire project has been built toward.

Why the other options are wrong

A. Genuinely current technology may enable on-site cannulation before transport, and this family's questions deserve honest, timely response, not deferral.

C. This specific status carries direct, particular relevance to determining candidacy, as detailed in the correct answer.

D. This family deserves honest, timely communication throughout this process, not deferral until after this procedure concludes.

E. This genuinely complex circumstance requires coordinated, multidisciplinary management, not a single specialist acting independently.

Board Alert This is the truly final question of Mock Exam 1, deliberately constructed to require synthesis of ECMO candidacy, genuinely current transport technology, coordinated technical management, and honest family communication together.

Score Tracker: Mock Examination 1

Record your score by section below, and note any specific topic you missed for targeted review.

Reflection Prompts

Which section — Foundations, Organ Systems, or Application — was genuinely your weakest? That section deserves your next block of revision time, not the section you already feel confident in.

For any question you missed, return to the specific chapter this content was drawn from and re-read that chapter's own closing synthesis for that subdomain.

Two further mock examinations follow this one. Space them out rather than taking all three in immediate succession — spaced repetition genuinely outperforms clustered review.

Mock Examination 2

A Second, Fully Independent Practice Examination

60 Questions — Foundations, Organ Systems, and Application Together

A Genuinely New Set of Vignettes

Every question in this exam is newly written and entirely independent of Mock Examination 1 — no clinical scenario, patient presentation, or specific correct answer is repeated. The same proportional structure applies: a foundations section drawing on Volume 1, a substantial organ systems section drawing on Volumes 2 and 3, and an application section drawing on Volume 4's surgical, transport, systems, ethical, and biostatistical content.

Where Mock Examination 1 tended to test a single, specific fact or connection per question, this second exam leans slightly more on connected, multi-step reasoning — a finding that requires recalling why it happens before deciding what to do about it, or a research finding that requires critical, methodological appraisal before its result can be trusted. This mirrors how difficulty tends to build across a genuine sequence of practice examinations.

How to Use This Exam

If you have already completed Mock Examination 1, leave at least several days between the two — spaced repetition is considerably more effective for long-term retention than immediate, back-to-back repetition.

Work through all 60 questions in a single, timed sitting if possible, targeting roughly 90 seconds per question.

Pay particular attention to any question you get wrong for a reason genuinely different from a similar question you missed in Mock Examination 1 — a repeated category of error is more diagnostic than an isolated one.

A Note on Figures

Every figure in this book is original artwork, drawn specifically for it. No stock images, no licensed photographs and no third-party illustrations are used anywhere in the text.

Questions

Section A: Foundations (Questions 1-9) — Section B: Organ Systems (Questions 10–58) — Section C: Application (Questions 59–60, and interspersed throughout Section B)

Question 1

A 26-week gestation infant is delivered via emergency caesarean section for significant placental abruption. At 60 seconds of life, heart rate is 50 beats per minute despite 30 seconds of effective positive pressure ventilation confirmed by chest rise. Which of the following represents the correct, immediate next step?

A. Continue positive pressure ventilation alone for a further, extended period before considering any additional intervention

B. Begin chest compressions coordinated with ventilation at a 3:1 ratio, since this heart rate remains below 60 despite 30 seconds of effective ventilation

C. Administer intravenous epinephrine immediately, without first initiating chest compressions

D. Discontinue resuscitative efforts entirely, given this infant's extremely preterm gestational age

E. Immediately clamp and cut the umbilical cord before any further, additional resuscitative step

Answer: B. With a heart rate below 60 despite 30 seconds of effective ventilation, chest compressions coordinated with ventilation at a 3:1 ratio represent the correct, immediate next step in this algorithm.

This vignette directly tests the sequential, escalating structure of the Neonatal Resuscitation Program algorithm: a heart rate below 60 despite 30 seconds of confirmed, effective positive pressure ventilation meets the specific, established threshold for initiating chest compressions.

Chest compressions are coordinated with ventilation at a 3:1 ratio, this specific, coordinated approach directly reflecting established, current resuscitation guidance rather than either intervention delivered in isolation.

Epinephrine is reserved for continued, significant bradycardia despite effective ventilation and compressions together — not indicated as an immediate step before chest compressions have genuinely been attempted.

Why the other options are wrong

A. This heart rate meets the specific threshold for chest compressions; continuing ventilation alone is not the correct, immediate step.

C. Epinephrine is reserved for continued bradycardia despite effective ventilation and compressions together, not before compressions.

D. This gestational age alone does not represent an indication to discontinue resuscitative efforts at this early stage.

E. Cord clamping timing is not the immediate priority; this heart rate requires immediate escalation to chest compressions.

Board Alert A heart rate below 60 despite 30 seconds of effective positive pressure ventilation meets the threshold for chest compressions, coordinated with ventilation at a 3:1 ratio.

Question 2

A 25-week gestation infant is 3 days old. An echocardiogram performed for a murmur incidentally demonstrates ongoing left ventricular diastolic function that has not yet reached its expected, mature pattern. Which of the following best explains the expected, current understanding of this infant's own cardiac maturational trajectory?

A. This infant's cardiac diastolic function has already achieved full, mature stability, making this described finding inaccurate

B. Genuinely current echocardiographic evidence demonstrates that left ventricular diastolic flow dynamics continue maturing for weeks after birth, with this specific parameter typically stabilising around 6 to 8 weeks of age, and intraventricular pressure differences continuing to increase until approximately 6 months of age

C. Cardiac maturation concludes entirely and abruptly at the moment of birth, with no genuine, further postnatal change of any kind

D. This specific finding carries no genuine relationship to this infant's own gestational age at birth

E. This infant's cardiac diastolic function will never achieve a genuinely mature, stable pattern regardless of postnatal age

Answer: B. Genuinely current echocardiographic evidence demonstrates that left ventricular diastolic flow dynamics continue maturing for weeks, typically stabilising around 6 to 8 weeks, with intraventricular pressure differences continuing to increase until approximately 6 months of age.

This vignette directly tests this book's own established physiology content regarding extended, ongoing cardiac maturation: circulatory and pulmonary physiological changes genuinely continue for a considerably extended period following birth, well beyond the immediate, dramatic transition this book has otherwise emphasised.

Genuinely current, quantified echocardiographic evidence demonstrates left ventricular diastolic flow dynamics stabilising at 6 to 8 weeks of postnatal age, with intraventricular pressure differences continuing to increase until approximately 6 months of age — a genuinely extended, ongoing maturational trajectory distinct from this infant's own dramatic, initial circulatory transition at birth.

This reflects this book's own repeated theme that neonatal physiological maturation genuinely, comprehensively extends across multiple, distinct organ systems over a genuinely extended timeline, well beyond the delivery room this book's opening content might otherwise seem to emphasise.

Why the other options are wrong

A. This infant's cardiac diastolic function genuinely remains in an ongoing maturational process at this early postnatal age.

C. Genuine, ongoing cardiac maturation continues for a considerably extended period following birth, not concluding abruptly at delivery.

D. This infant's own gestational age carries direct, genuine relevance to this ongoing maturational trajectory.

E. This function will genuinely, eventually achieve a mature, stable pattern, typically by approximately 6 to 8 weeks of age.

Board Alert Left ventricular diastolic flow dynamics stabilise at 6–8 weeks postnatal age; intraventricular pressure differences continue increasing until approximately 6 months — cardiac maturation genuinely extends well beyond birth.

Question 3

A 30-week gestation infant develops significant hypotension on day 1 of life that has responded poorly to two sequential normal saline boluses. The clinical team is considering the underlying reason for this limited fluid responsiveness. Which of the following best explains this infant's own limited response to volume alone?

A. This infant's myocardium demonstrates an identical response to increased preload as a term or adult myocardium, making fluid responsiveness equally reliable

B. This infant's genuinely immature myocardium, carrying reduced myofibrillar content, demonstrates a genuinely limited Frank-Starling reserve, meaning fluid administration alone frequently provides more limited haemodynamic benefit than in a more mature myocardium, supporting active consideration of vasopressor or inotropic support alongside continued, careful fluid assessment

C. This infant's hypotension is entirely unrelated to any genuine, underlying cardiac physiological consideration

D. Increased afterload carries no genuine relevance to this infant's own cardiac function of any kind

E. This infant's limited response to fluid boluses indicates that no further, active intervention of any kind is genuinely warranted

---

Answer: B. **This infant's genuinely immature myocardium, with reduced myofibrillar content, demonstrates a genuinely limited Frank-Starling reserve, meaning fluid alone provides more limited benefit — supporting active consideration of vasopressor or inotropic support.**

This vignette directly tests this book's own three-part myocardial immaturity framework: reduced myofibrillar content structurally explains a genuinely limited preload response through the Frank-Starling mechanism, meaning aggressive fluid administration alone may provide genuinely more limited haemodynamic benefit than in the considerably more preload-responsive, mature myocardium.

This same, immature myocardium also demonstrates genuinely elevated sensitivity to increased afterload and genuinely important reliance on heart rate for compensation, together forming a complete, three-part framework directly relevant to correctly, safely managing significant hypotension in this exact population.

This reflects this book's own repeated theme that correctly, safely treating this common, genuinely important condition requires actively applying this same, foundational myocardial framework, rather than assuming an identical management approach directly transferred from the mature, adult heart.

Why the other options are wrong

A. This infant's myocardium demonstrates a genuinely limited, not identical, response to increased preload compared with a mature heart.

C. This hypotension carries direct, genuine relevance to this infant's own underlying cardiac physiology, as detailed in the correct answer.

D. Afterload sensitivity carries direct, genuine relevance to this infant's own cardiac function, as detailed in the correct answer.

E. Active, further intervention, including consideration of vasopressor or inotropic support, remains genuinely warranted.

Board Alert The immature myocardium's reduced myofibrillar content produces a genuinely limited Frank-Starling reserve, meaning fluid boluses alone often provide limited benefit — supporting active consideration of vasopressor or inotropic support.

Question 4

A 32-week gestation infant on postnatal day 4 has a blood gas showing pH 7.18, PCO_2 40 mmHg, and a significantly reduced bicarbonate for gestational age. Which of the following best reflects the correct, immediate interpretation and next step for this specific finding?

A. This blood gas reflects a primary respiratory disturbance requiring immediate ventilator escalation alone

B. This blood gas reflects a primary metabolic disturbance, and given this book's own established, current association between metabolic acidosis occurring within the first 72 hours of life and significant intraventricular haemorrhage, this finding should prompt active, structured evaluation for an underlying cause, such as significant hypoperfusion, rather than reflexive bicarbonate administration alone

C. This finding carries no genuine, connected relevance to this infant's own neurological status of any kind

D. Sodium bicarbonate should genuinely, immediately be administered as the correct, first-line, and complete response to this specific finding

E. This specific finding requires no further, active clinical evaluation of any kind

Answer: B. **This blood gas reflects a primary metabolic disturbance, and given the established association between early metabolic acidosis and significant intraventricular haemorrhage, this finding should prompt active evaluation for an underlying cause rather than reflexive bicarbonate administration.**

This vignette directly tests this book's own foundational acid-base classification: a normal PCO2 with significantly reduced bicarbonate reflects a primary metabolic, rather than respiratory, disturbance — the classification principle directly determining the correct, appropriate diagnostic and management approach.

This book's own genuinely current, honest content directly establishes that metabolic acidosis specifically, occurring within the first 72 hours of life, carries a specific, established association with significant intraventricular haemorrhage, meaning this specific finding on day 4 warrants active, prompt clinical attention and structured evaluation for an underlying cause.

Correctly, actively identifying the specific underlying cause — significant hypoperfusion and lactic acidosis, significant renal bicarbonate loss, or another connected cause — directly determines the appropriate, targeted treatment this finding genuinely requires, since correcting the acidosis alone without addressing this same, underlying cause provides genuinely limited, temporary benefit.

Why the other options are wrong

A. This finding reflects a primary metabolic, not respiratory, disturbance; ventilator escalation alone is not the correct approach.

C. This finding carries direct, established, connected relevance to neurological risk, as detailed in the correct answer.

D. Correcting the underlying cause, not reflexive bicarbonate administration alone, represents the correct, complete approach.

E. Active, structured clinical evaluation is genuinely warranted for this specific finding.

Board Alert Metabolic acidosis within the first 72 hours of life carries an established association with significant intraventricular haemorrhage — correctly identifying and treating the underlying cause, not reflexive bicarbonate alone, is the correct approach.

Question 5

A 26-week gestation infant is receiving midazolam by continuous infusion for sedation. The clinical team is considering administering a bolus dose in combination with a fentanyl bolus for an upcoming procedure. Which of the following best reflects the correct, safety-relevant consideration for this specific combination?

A. This specific combination carries no genuine, connected safety consideration of any kind

B. Midazolam's own genuinely delayed elimination in the neonatal period carries particular, genuine caution when this medication is administered as a bolus injection or combined with a specific opioid, given this specific combination's own genuine, established, associated hypotension risk

C. Bolus administration of either medication carries an identical safety profile to continuous, gradual infusion in every specific circumstance

D. This infant's own gestational age carries no genuine relevance to correctly, safely administering either of these two medications

E. This specific combination should genuinely, always be avoided in every circumstance, regardless of clinical indication

Answer: B. **Midazolam's genuinely delayed neonatal elimination carries particular caution when administered as a bolus or combined with a specific opioid, given this combination's own genuine, established, associated hypotension risk.**

This vignette directly tests this book's own established pharmacology content regarding midazolam's own genuinely distinctive developmental pharmacokinetics: this specific medication's own genuinely prolonged half-life in this population directly carries genuine, specific implication for correctly, safely titrating and monitoring this specific sedative agent.

Genuine, specific caution is particularly warranted when this specific medication is administered as a bolus injection, rather than a genuinely gradual, continuous infusion, or when genuinely combined with a specific opioid medication, given this specific combination's own genuine, established, associated hypotension risk.

This reflects this book's own repeated theme that correctly, precisely understanding a specific medication's own genuine, developmentally distinctive pharmacokinetics directly informs safe, correct clinical administration technique, rather than assuming bolus and infusion administration carry an identical safety profile.

Why the other options are wrong

A. A genuine, specific safety consideration exists, as detailed in the correct answer, not an absence of connected concern.

C. Bolus administration carries a genuinely different, elevated risk profile compared with gradual, continuous infusion.

D. This infant's own gestational age carries direct, genuine relevance to safely administering these medications.

E. This combination is not universally, categorically avoided, but rather requires particular, active caution as detailed in the correct answer.

Board Alert Midazolam's genuinely delayed neonatal elimination requires particular caution with bolus administration or combination with a specific opioid, given the genuine, established, associated hypotension risk.

Question 6

A 24-week gestation infant has been receiving caffeine citrate for apnoea of prematurity since day 1 of life and is now 6 weeks old. The family asks about this medication's own longer-term effect on this infant's development. Which of the following best reflects the correct, honest, current understanding of this specific question?

A. Caffeine carries no genuine, established relationship to this infant's own neurodevelopmental outcome of any kind

B. Genuinely current research has specifically demonstrated that cumulative caffeine exposure, rather than any single, isolated dose, directly predicts this infant's own longer-term neurodevelopmental outcome, meaning correctly, completely evaluating this medication's own genuine, longer-term effect requires actively tracking total, accumulated exposure across this infant's own entire treatment course

C. A single, isolated caffeine dose provides an entirely complete, sufficient picture of this medication's own eventual, longer-term effect

D. This specific question deserves no genuine, substantive, honest response of any kind

E. Caffeine's own longer-term developmental effect has been definitively, completely, and uniformly established with no genuine, remaining uncertainty of any kind

Answer: B. Genuinely current research demonstrates that cumulative caffeine exposure, rather than any single, isolated dose, directly predicts longer-term neurodevelopmental outcome, requiring active tracking of total, accumulated exposure.

This vignette directly tests this book's own genuinely current, honest pharmacology content: genuinely current research has specifically demonstrated that cumulative caffeine exposure, rather than any single, isolated dose considered alone, directly predicts a given infant's own longer-term neurodevelopmental outcome.

This means correctly, completely evaluating this specific medication's own genuine, longer-term effect requires actively tracking total, accumulated exposure across this infant's own entire treatment course, rather than any single, isolated measurement or dose considered in complete isolation.

This reflects this book's own repeated theme, established for other genuinely important, significant exposures, that cumulative, rather than isolated, exposure frequently carries the more genuinely important predictive relevance, supporting an honest, complete response to this family's genuine question rather than a dismissive or falsely certain answer.

Why the other options are wrong

A. A direct, established relationship exists between this medication and neurodevelopmental outcome, as detailed in the correct answer.

C. Cumulative exposure, not a single, isolated dose, provides the genuinely more complete, predictive picture.

D. This specific question deserves a genuine, substantive, honest response, as detailed in the correct answer.

E. Genuine, remaining nuance exists regarding this specific relationship, requiring the honest, complete response detailed in the correct answer.

> **Board Alert** Genuinely current research demonstrates that cumulative caffeine exposure, rather than any single, isolated dose, directly predicts longer-term neurodevelopmental outcome.

Question 7

A 22-week gestation fetus is diagnosed with a significant, isolated structural anomaly considered life-limiting. The family expresses a genuine wish to continue the pregnancy and pursue perinatal palliative care. Which of the following best reflects the correct, complete understanding of this specific pathway?

- **A.** Perinatal palliative care represents a genuinely inferior, lesser pathway compared with active resuscitation in every specific circumstance
- **B.** Offering perinatal palliative care to this family should genuinely be seen as an opportunity to further, rather than limit, this same family's own genuine autonomy and beneficent, complete care, precisely paralleling this same family's own equally genuine right to choose termination or active resuscitation instead
- **C.** This family's own genuine wish carries no genuine relevance to correctly determining this infant's own appropriate care pathway
- **D.** Perinatal palliative care requires no genuine, structured, coordinated planning of any kind
- **E.** This family should genuinely be discouraged from pursuing this specific pathway, regardless of their own expressed preference

> **Answer: B. Offering perinatal palliative care should be seen as an opportunity to further, rather than limit, this family's own genuine autonomy and beneficent care, precisely paralleling their equally genuine right to choose termination or active resuscitation instead.**
>
> This vignette directly tests this book's own foundational ethics content: perinatal palliative care represents one, specific option along a genuinely broader spectrum of care, this same spectrum also genuinely including pregnancy termination and full, active neonatal resuscitation and treatment together.
>
> Correctly, actively supporting a family's own genuine choice to continue a

pregnancy following a significant, life-limiting diagnosis directly connects to the genuine autonomy principle established throughout this book, meaning offering perinatal palliative care to a family genuinely making this choice should genuinely be seen as an opportunity to further, rather than limit, this same family's own genuine autonomy.

A genuinely coordinated, structured birth plan directly extends this book's own antenatal counselling content, allowing this family's own genuine values and goals to be clearly, explicitly documented and honoured throughout this infant's own entire, anticipated clinical course.

Why the other options are wrong

A. Perinatal palliative care represents a genuinely legitimate, equal option, not an inferior pathway, as detailed in the correct answer.

C. This family's own genuine wish carries direct, essential relevance to determining this infant's own appropriate care pathway.

D. This specific pathway genuinely requires structured, coordinated planning, as detailed in the correct answer.

E. This family's own expressed preference should genuinely be respected and supported, not actively discouraged.

Board Alert Offering perinatal palliative care should be seen as an opportunity to further, not limit, a family's genuine autonomy — precisely paralleling their equally genuine right to choose termination or active resuscitation instead.

Question 8

A term infant presents with significant hypotonia, macroglossia, omphalocele, and significant hypoglycaemia in the first day of life. Which of the following best explains the most likely, underlying diagnosis and its own connected significance?

A. This combination of findings carries no genuine, connected, underlying diagnosis of any kind

B. This presentation is highly consistent with Beckwith-Wiedemann syndrome, a specific overgrowth syndrome directly explaining this connected combination of findings, and this diagnosis carries genuine, established relevance to this infant's own subsequent risk of specific embryonal tumours, supporting active, structured surveillance

C. Macroglossia in this specific context carries no genuine, diagnostic significance of any kind

D. This presentation should be managed without any further, active diagnostic evaluation or subsequent surveillance of any kind

E. This infant's hypoglycaemia is entirely unrelated to this infant's own other, connected findings

Answer: B. **This presentation is highly consistent with Beckwith-Wiedemann syndrome, directly explaining this connected combination of findings, and this diagnosis carries genuine, established relevance to subsequent embryonal tumour risk, supporting active, structured surveillance.**

This vignette presents the classic, connected combination for Beckwith-Wiedemann syndrome: macroglossia, omphalocele, and significant hypoglycaemia together reflect this specific overgrowth syndrome's own characteristic, connected pattern of findings.

This connected reasoning — recognising that a single, underlying genetic and developmental mechanism directly explains multiple, apparently distinct findings together — represents exactly the kind of mechanism-first, cross-system diagnostic reasoning this book has modelled throughout its own genetics content.

This specific diagnosis carries genuine, established relevance to this infant's own subsequent, elevated risk of specific embryonal tumours, including Wilms tumour and hepatoblastoma, directly supporting active, structured surveillance extending well beyond this infant's own immediate, neonatal presentation.

Why the other options are wrong

A. A specific, connected, underlying diagnosis directly explains this combination of findings, as detailed in the correct answer.

C. This specific finding carries direct, diagnostic significance in this connected presentation.

D. Active, structured diagnostic evaluation and subsequent surveillance are genuinely warranted for this specific presentation.

E. This infant's hypoglycaemia is directly, mechanistically connected to this same, underlying diagnosis.

Board Alert Macroglossia, omphalocele, and significant hypoglycaemia together suggest Beckwith-Wiedemann syndrome, carrying genuine, established relevance to subsequent embryonal tumour risk requiring active surveillance.

Question 9

A 25-week gestation infant is 2 weeks old and has completed an initial course of indomethacin for a haemodynamically significant patent ductus arteriosus. The clinical team is now considering a second course. Which of the following best reflects a genuinely important, connected safety consideration for this specific medication?

A. This medication carries no genuine, established relationship to renal function of any kind

B. This medication, particularly with prolonged or repeated use, carries genuine, established renal risk, directly connecting to this book's own established content regarding prenatal indomethacin exposure and fetal ductal and renal risk, meaning correctly, safely considering a second course requires active, careful attention to this infant's own current renal status

C. This medication carries an identical safety profile regardless of the specific number of courses administered

D. Renal status carries no genuine relevance to correctly considering repeated administration of this specific medication

E. This medication should genuinely, always be readministered without any further, active safety consideration of any kind

Answer: B. This medication carries genuine, established renal risk with prolonged or repeated use, directly connecting to this book's content on prenatal indomethacin exposure — requiring careful attention to renal status before a second course.

This vignette directly tests this book's own established pharmacology and maternal-fetal medicine content together: maternal indomethacin exposure carries specific, established fetal ductal and renal risk when used prolonged or beyond a specific gestational threshold, this same medication's prostaglandin-inhibiting mechanism directly relevant to postnatal administration as well.

This same, connected mechanism directly informs correctly, safely considering repeated, postnatal administration: this medication's own genuine, established renal risk, particularly with prolonged or repeated use, requires active, careful attention to this infant's own current renal status before proceeding with a further course.

This reflects this book's own repeated theme that a specific medication's own genuine, connected risk profile, established in one specific clinical context, frequently carries direct, connected relevance to this same medication's own further, related clinical application.

Why the other options are wrong

A. A direct, established relationship exists between this medication and renal function, as detailed in the correct answer.

C. Repeated or prolonged use carries a genuinely different, elevated risk profile compared with a single, initial course.

D. Renal status carries direct, essential relevance to considering repeated administration, as detailed in the correct answer.

E. Active, careful safety consideration is genuinely required before readministering this specific medication.

Board Alert Indomethacin carries genuine, established renal risk, particularly with prolonged or repeated use, requiring careful attention to current renal status before considering a further course.

Mock Exam 2 — Section B: Organ Systems | Universal Task 3: Diagnosis, Testing and Monitoring

Question 10

A 33-week gestation infant develops significant respiratory distress at 2 hours of life. A chest radiograph shows low lung volumes with diffuse, fine granular opacities and air bronchograms extending to the periphery. Which of the following represents the most appropriate, immediate management step?

A. Immediate discharge home, since this presentation is entirely benign and self-limited

B. This presentation is highly consistent with respiratory distress syndrome reflecting surfactant deficiency, and administration of exogenous surfactant, together with appropriate respiratory support, represents the correct, immediate management approach

C. This presentation requires immediate, empiric broad-spectrum antifungal therapy alone

D. This presentation should be managed exclusively with intravenous fluid restriction, without any specific respiratory intervention

E. This specific radiographic pattern carries no genuine relationship to any specific, established neonatal respiratory diagnosis

Answer: B. **This presentation — low lung volumes, diffuse fine granular opacities, and air bronchograms — is highly consistent with surfactant-deficient respiratory distress syndrome, requiring exogenous surfactant administration and appropriate respiratory support.**

This vignette presents the classic radiographic pattern of respiratory distress syndrome: low lung volumes, a diffuse, fine granular ('ground glass') opacification, and air bronchograms extending to the lung periphery, directly reflecting surfactant deficiency's own characteristic pathophysiology.

Correct, immediate management directly requires exogenous surfactant administration, this specific intervention directly addressing the underlying surfactant deficiency this presentation reflects, together with appropriate, structured respiratory support tailored to this infant's own specific, ongoing needs.

This distinguishes this presentation from transient tachypnoea of the newborn, which typically demonstrates a genuinely different, streaky pattern with fluid in the interlobar fissures and a considerably more favourable, self-limited course without specific surfactant intervention.

Why the other options are wrong

A. This presentation requires active respiratory management, not immediate discharge as though entirely benign.

C. This presentation is consistent with surfactant deficiency, not a fungal infection requiring antifungal therapy.

D. Specific respiratory intervention, including surfactant administration, is required, not fluid restriction alone.

E. This specific radiographic pattern carries direct, established relevance to respiratory distress syndrome.

Board Alert Respiratory distress syndrome: low lung volumes, diffuse fine granular opacities, air bronchograms. Treat with exogenous surfactant and appropriate respiratory support.

Question 11

A 28-week gestation infant on day 8 of life has genuinely current NEC surgical guideline recommendations under consideration by the surgical and neonatology teams, following confirmed pneumatosis intestinalis without pneumoperitoneum. Which of the following best reflects the correct, honest interpretation of the current evidence base guiding this specific decision?

A. Every specific recommendation regarding surgical timing in this circumstance carries entirely high, definitively established certainty of evidence

B. Genuinely current guideline evidence honestly acknowledges (very) low certainty of evidence for the great majority of specific recommendations regarding surgical timing short of pneumoperitoneum, meaning this decision genuinely requires dynamic, individualised clinical assessment rather than a single, universally validated threshold

C. This specific finding carries no genuine relationship to any established surgical decision-making framework

D. A universally validated threshold for surgical timing in this exact circumstance has already been definitively established

E. This infant's own clinical trajectory carries no genuine relevance to this specific surgical timing decision

Answer: B. **Genuinely current guideline evidence honestly acknowledges (very) low certainty for most recommendations regarding surgical timing short of pneumoperitoneum, requiring dynamic, individualised assessment rather than a single, validated threshold.**

This vignette directly tests this book's own established surgical content: beyond the single, unambiguous pneumoperitoneum finding, no genuinely universal, validated threshold or specific criteria currently exist for reliably identifying which specific infants may be genuinely 'failing medical management.'

This chapter's own genuinely current guideline honestly, transparently acknowledges (very) low certainty of evidence for the great majority of its own specific recommendations, this specific, honest acknowledgement reflecting the guideline development panel's own transparent, systematic grading of the actual, underlying evidence base.

This means correctly, safely deciding whether and precisely when to proceed to surgery in this specific circumstance genuinely requires dynamic, individualised clinical assessment, actively integrating laboratory markers and targeted imaging together, rather than a single, reliable, validated decision rule.

Why the other options are wrong

A. Genuine, low certainty exists for most recommendations, as detailed in the correct answer, not universally high certainty.

C. This finding has direct, established relevance to this surgical decision-making framework, as detailed in the correct answer.

D. No genuinely universal, validated threshold currently exists short of pneumoperitoneum, as detailed in the correct answer.

E. This infant's own clinical trajectory carries direct, genuine relevance to this specific decision.

Board Alert Genuinely current NEC surgical guideline evidence honestly acknowledges (very) low certainty for most recommendations short of pneumoperitoneum, requiring dynamic, individualised clinical assessment.

Question 12

A term infant develops significant respiratory distress, a scaphoid chest, and asymmetric breath sounds with a shifted cardiac apex within the first hours of life. A chest radiograph confirms a large pneumothorax. Which of the following represents the most appropriate, immediate management step?

A. Observation alone, without any active, specific intervention, since pneumothorax in the neonate always, universally resolves spontaneously without treatment

B. Given this infant's significant respiratory distress and radiographically confirmed, large pneumothorax, needle decompression or chest tube placement represents the correct, immediate, active intervention

C. This presentation requires immediate, empiric antibiotic therapy alone, without any specific respiratory intervention

D. This specific finding carries no genuine urgency of any kind, regardless of this infant's own degree of respiratory distress

E. This infant should genuinely receive positive pressure ventilation via face mask alone, without any further, specific evaluation

Answer: B. Given significant respiratory distress with a radiographically confirmed, large pneumothorax, needle decompression or chest tube placement represents the correct, immediate, active intervention.

This vignette presents a significant, symptomatic pneumothorax: significant respiratory distress, asymmetric breath sounds, and cardiac apex shift together directly reflect a genuinely significant accumulation of pleural air under tension, requiring active, immediate intervention rather than passive observation.

Correct, immediate management directly requires active decompression, either through needle aspiration for rapid, initial relief or chest tube placement for definitive, ongoing management, this specific intervention directly addressing the genuine, immediate physiological compromise this presentation reflects.

This reflects this book's own repeated theme that correctly, rapidly recognising a specific, connected, and genuinely urgent clinical pattern directly changes the appropriate, immediate management approach, rather than assuming passive, watchful observation is universally appropriate regardless of clinical severity.

Why the other options are wrong

A. A significant, symptomatic pneumothorax requires active intervention, not universal, passive observation alone.

C. Active respiratory decompression, not antibiotic therapy alone, represents the correct, immediate intervention.

D. This specific finding carries genuine, significant urgency given this infant's own degree of respiratory distress.

E. Active decompression, not face mask ventilation alone, represents the correct, immediate approach to this specific finding.

Board Alert A significant, symptomatic pneumothorax with respiratory distress and mediastinal shift requires active, immediate decompression — needle aspiration or chest tube placement — not passive observation.

Question 13

A 24-week gestation infant is 3 weeks old and remains on mechanical ventilation. The clinical team notes that this infant's own head circumference has crossed downward across two major percentile lines over the past 2 weeks. Which of the following best reflects the correct, active response to this specific finding?

A. This finding carries no genuine, connected significance of any kind, requiring no further, active evaluation

B. This finding warrants active, prompt evaluation, including cranial ultrasound, given this specific pattern's own genuine, established association with connected neurological injury and its own genuine relevance to this infant's own longer-term neurodevelopmental trajectory

C. This finding should genuinely be attributed exclusively to normal, expected growth variation, without any further, active consideration

D. Head circumference measurement carries no genuine, established relevance to this infant's own neurological status of any kind

E. This finding requires no further, structured, longer-term follow-up of any kind

Answer: B. **This finding warrants active, prompt evaluation including cranial ultrasound, given its genuine, established association with connected neurological injury and relevance to longer-term neurodevelopmental trajectory.**

This vignette directly tests this book's own established neurology content: a significant, declining head circumference trajectory carries genuine, connected significance, since this specific pattern can reflect significant, underlying neurological injury or evolving, connected pathology.

This same finding directly warrants active, prompt evaluation, including cranial ultrasound, to actively assess for a specific, underlying cause, reflecting this book's own repeated theme that a specific, quantifiable clinical trend, correctly and actively monitored, frequently provides genuinely important, connected diagnostic information.

This same finding directly supports this book's own established, structured, longer-term neurodevelopmental follow-up programme, extending clinical attention well beyond the immediate, acute period, given this specific finding's own genuine, connected relevance to this infant's own longer-term developmental trajectory.

Why the other options are wrong

A. This finding carries genuine, connected significance, warranting active evaluation, not an absence of relevance.

C. This finding warrants active evaluation for a specific, underlying cause, not automatic attribution to normal variation.

D. A direct, established relevance exists between this measurement and neurological status, as detailed in the correct answer.

E. This finding supports structured, longer-term follow-up, as detailed in the correct answer.

Board Alert A significantly declining head circumference trajectory warrants active, prompt evaluation including cranial ultrasound, given established association with connected neurological injury.

Question 14

A 29-week gestation infant is 10 days old and has been advancing enteral feeds using the mother's own expressed milk. The clinical team is discussing the specific timing for initiating human milk fortification. Which of the following best reflects the correct, evidence-based consideration for this specific decision?

A. Fortification should never genuinely be initiated at any specific point during this infant's own hospitalisation

B. Fortification timing requires active, individualised clinical judgment, generally initiated once feeds have reached a specific, established volume threshold demonstrating genuine feeding tolerance, reflecting this population's own genuinely elevated nutritional requirements balanced against genuine, connected feeding tolerance considerations

C. Fortification should genuinely, always be initiated on the very first day of any enteral feeding, regardless of this infant's own specific, individual tolerance

D. This infant's own specific feeding tolerance carries no genuine relevance to correctly timing this specific intervention

E. This specific decision carries no genuine, established evidence base of any kind

Answer: B. Fortification timing requires active, individualised clinical judgment, generally initiated once feeds reach an established volume threshold demonstrating genuine tolerance, balancing elevated nutritional requirements against feeding tolerance considerations.

This vignette directly tests this book's own established nutrition content: human milk fortification is generally required to meet the elevated protein, calcium, phosphorus, and caloric requirements of the preterm infant, since unfortified human milk alone typically does not provide sufficient quantities of these specific nutrients.

Correctly, individually timing this specific intervention requires active clinical judgment, generally initiated once feeds have reached a specific, established volume threshold demonstrating genuine feeding tolerance, rather than either universal avoidance or reflexive, immediate initiation regardless of this infant's own individual, connected tolerance.

This reflects this book's own repeated theme that correctly, individually tailoring nutritional support to this population's own genuinely distinctive requirements requires active, balanced clinical judgment considering both this infant's own elevated nutritional need and this same infant's own genuine, individual feeding tolerance together.

Why the other options are wrong

A. Fortification is generally appropriate and beneficial in this population, not universally avoided at every point.

C. Individualised timing based on genuine tolerance, not universal, immediate initiation regardless of tolerance, is correct.

D. This infant's own feeding tolerance carries direct, essential relevance to correctly timing this specific intervention.

E. This specific decision carries direct, established evidence base, as detailed in the correct answer.

Board Alert Human milk fortification timing requires individualised clinical judgment, generally initiated once feeds reach an established volume threshold demonstrating genuine feeding tolerance.

Question 15

A term infant develops significant respiratory distress and cyanosis that fails to improve significantly with supplemental oxygen. An echocardiogram confirms transposition of the great arteries. Which of the following best explains why this infant's own cyanosis persists despite oxygen administration?

A. Supplemental oxygen administration carries no genuine, established relationship to cyanosis of any kind in this specific condition

B. This condition reflects parallel, rather than properly connected, systemic and pulmonary circulations, meaning oxygenated blood returning from the lungs continues recirculating through the pulmonary circuit alone, while deoxygenated systemic blood continues recirculating systemically, largely independent of inspired oxygen concentration, unless genuine mixing occurs through a connected shunt

C. This infant's cyanosis reflects a primary pulmonary parenchymal disease process entirely unrelated to this confirmed cardiac diagnosis

D. This specific condition requires no further, active management of any kind beyond supplemental oxygen alone

E. Genuine mixing between these two circulations carries no genuine relevance to this infant's own oxygenation status

Answer: B. **Transposition of the great arteries reflects parallel, disconnected systemic and pulmonary circulations, meaning oxygenated and deoxygenated blood each continue recirculating separately, largely independent of inspired oxygen, unless genuine mixing occurs through a connected shunt.**

This vignette directly tests foundational, connected cardiac physiology: in transposition of the great arteries, the aorta arises from the right ventricle and the pulmonary artery from the left ventricle, creating two, genuinely parallel, rather than properly connected, circulations.

This means oxygenated blood returning from the lungs continues recirculating through the pulmonary circuit alone, while deoxygenated systemic blood continues recirculating systemically, this specific, parallel arrangement directly explaining why supplemental oxygen alone provides genuinely limited benefit, since this intervention cannot correct this fundamental, structural circulatory problem.

Correct management requires actively establishing genuine mixing between these two, parallel circulations, whether through a patent ductus arteriosus, a patent foramen ovale, or an urgent balloon atrial septostomy, directly reflecting this book's own repeated theme that a specific, structural cardiac lesion frequently requires targeted, structural intervention rather than supportive measures alone.

Why the other options are wrong

A. A direct, mechanistic relationship exists between oxygen administration and this specific condition's own limited response.

C. This cyanosis reflects this confirmed, structural cardiac lesion, not a primary, unrelated pulmonary process.

D. Active, further, targeted management, beyond supplemental oxygen alone, is genuinely required for this specific condition.

E. A direct, essential relationship exists between genuine mixing and this infant's own oxygenation status.

Board Alert Transposition of the great arteries creates parallel, disconnected circulations; supplemental oxygen alone provides limited benefit. Correct management requires establishing genuine mixing between these two circuits.

Question 16

A 26-week gestation infant develops significant, new-onset abdominal distension and bloody stools on day 14 of life. Given the genuinely current 2026 randomised trial evidence this book has established, which of the following best reflects a genuinely current, active area of research directly relevant to correctly timing surgical intervention in this specific circumstance?

A. No genuinely current, active research exists regarding correctly timing surgical intervention in necrotising enterocolitis

B. A genuinely current, specific randomised controlled trial has directly compared traditional Bell's criteria against a specific, further strategy combining metabolic disorder components with positive paracentesis, finding this further, combined strategy directly associated with earlier surgery and better outcomes for perforation, intestinal necrosis, and reoperation

C. This genuinely current research finding carries no genuine relevance to correctly timing surgical intervention in this specific circumstance

D. Paracentesis carries a genuine, significant complication risk directly attributed to this specific procedure itself, according to this genuinely current trial

E. Traditional Bell's criteria have already been definitively, completely replaced by universal, current consensus

Answer: B. A genuinely current, specific 2026 randomised trial directly compared traditional Bell's criteria against a combined metabolic-disorder-plus-paracentesis strategy, finding this combined strategy associated with earlier surgery and better outcomes.

This vignette directly tests this book's own genuinely current necrotising enterocolitis content: a genuinely current, specific randomised controlled trial, published in 2026 and enrolling 117 preterm neonates with confirmed surgical necrotising enterocolitis, has directly compared traditional Bell's criteria against a specific, further strategy combining metabolic disorder components with positive paracentesis.

This genuinely current trial found this further, combined strategy directly associated with earlier surgery and better, measurably improved outcomes for perforation, intestinal necrosis, and reoperation, with no specific complications directly attributed to the paracentesis procedure itself.

This reflects this book's own repeated theme regarding genuinely current, active research directly attempting to bring greater, evidence-based structure to this genuinely uncertain surgical decision-making landscape, even as the broader, universal threshold this book has established genuinely remains elusive.

Why the other options are wrong

A. Genuinely current, active research exists, as detailed in the correct answer, not an absence of this research.

C. This research finding carries direct, genuine relevance to correctly timing surgical intervention, as detailed in the correct answer.

D. No specific complications were directly attributed to this procedure itself, according to this genuinely current trial.

E. This reflects an ongoing, active area of comparison, not a definitively completed replacement of traditional criteria.

Board Alert A genuinely current 2026 randomised trial compared traditional Bell's criteria against a combined metabolic-disorder-plus-paracentesis strategy, finding the combined strategy associated with earlier surgery and better outcomes.

Question 17

A term infant is noted to have a significant, single palmar crease, upslanting palpebral fissures, and significant hypotonia. An echocardiogram reveals a complete atrioventricular septal defect. Which of the following genetic diagnoses is most strongly suggested by this specific, connected combination of findings?

A. This combination of findings carries no genuine, connected relationship to any specific genetic diagnosis of any kind

B. This presentation is highly suggestive of trisomy 21, given this specific, connected combination of characteristic dysmorphic features together with a cardiac lesion carrying a well-established, elevated association with this specific chromosomal abnormality

C. This presentation is more consistent with trisomy 18, a condition carrying a considerably more severe, connected pattern of findings than described here

D. This specific cardiac lesion carries no genuine, established association with any specific chromosomal abnormality

E. Hypotonia in this specific context carries no genuine, diagnostic significance of any kind

Answer: B. This presentation is highly suggestive of trisomy 21, given this connected combination of characteristic dysmorphic features together with a cardiac lesion — complete atrioventricular septal defect — carrying a well-established, elevated association with this chromosomal abnormality.

This vignette presents the classic, connected combination for trisomy 21: a single palmar crease, upslanting palpebral fissures, and significant hypotonia together represent characteristic, connected dysmorphic features this book has established at length throughout its own genetics content.

The complete atrioventricular septal defect directly reinforces this specific diagnosis, this specific cardiac lesion carrying a well-established, particularly elevated association with trisomy 21 among the broader range of cardiac anomalies this same chromosomal abnormality can produce.

This connected reasoning — recognising that three or more minor anomalies together significantly increase the probability of an underlying, connected major anomaly or genetic syndrome, this book's own established, foundational dysmorphology principle — directly supports active, prompt genetic confirmation in this specific, connected presentation.

Why the other options are wrong

A. A direct, well-established, connected relationship exists between this combination and a specific genetic diagnosis.

C. This presentation, while requiring active differentiation, is more classically, specifically associated with trisomy 21 given this exact combination.

D. A direct, well-established, elevated association exists between this specific cardiac lesion and trisomy 21.

E. This specific finding carries direct, diagnostic significance in this connected presentation.

Board Alert A single palmar crease, upslanting palpebral fissures, hypotonia, and a complete atrioventricular septal defect together are highly suggestive of trisomy 21, given this cardiac lesion's well-established, elevated association.

Question 18

A 27-week gestation infant has genuinely current 2025 guideline recommendations under consideration for structured, longer-term follow-up. Which of the following best reflects this book's own established, correct understanding of this specific programme's own genuine scope?

A. Structured, longer-term follow-up is relevant exclusively to a single, specific high-risk population, with no genuine, broader, shared applicability across other, connected populations

B. This same, structured, longer-term follow-up principle directly reflects the same, shared surveillance principle this book has established repeatedly for other genuinely important, high-risk neonatal populations, regardless of which specific condition originates their own, particular elevated risk

C. Structured, longer-term follow-up carries no genuine, established relevance to this infant's own eventual outcome of any kind

D. This specific programme requires no genuine, coordinated, multidisciplinary involvement of any kind

E. This infant's own extreme prematurity carries no genuine relevance to correctly determining the need for this specific programme

Answer: B. Structured, longer-term follow-up directly reflects the same, shared surveillance principle this book establishes repeatedly for other high-risk populations, regardless of which specific condition originates their elevated risk.

This vignette directly tests this book's own repeated, cross-chapter demonstration: correctly, actively coordinating a specific, genuinely current, structured follow-up guideline with the extensive neurodevelopmental follow-up content established throughout this book for other genuinely important neonatal populations directly reflects a shared, structural principle.

This same, structured principle applies regardless of which specific, acute condition or intervention this population's own particular, elevated risk actually originates from, reinforcing this book's repeated, closing theme that a genuinely important, structural clinical principle established at length throughout this book continues to carry direct, connected relevance across the whole of neonatal medicine.

This reflects this book's own repeated theme that a specific, high-risk population's own longer-term, connected developmental trajectory requires the same, structured surveillance principle, whether this population's own elevated risk originates from extreme prematurity, hypoxic-ischaemic encephalopathy, ECMO support, or another connected, high-risk circumstance.

Why the other options are wrong

A. This principle carries genuine, broader, shared applicability across multiple populations, not exclusive relevance to a single population.

C. A direct, established relevance exists between this follow-up and this infant's own eventual outcome.

D. This specific programme genuinely requires coordinated, multidisciplinary involvement.

E. This infant's own extreme prematurity carries direct, genuine relevance to determining the need for this specific programme.

Board Alert Structured, longer-term neurodevelopmental follow-up reflects the same, shared surveillance principle across multiple high-risk populations, regardless of which specific condition originates their elevated risk.

Question 19

A 31-week gestation infant develops a significant, new-onset seizure on day 3 of life. Blood glucose is significantly low at 18 mg/dL. Which of the following represents the most appropriate, immediate next step?

A. No specific, immediate intervention is required, since this infant's seizure is unrelated to this same infant's own concurrently, significantly low glucose

B. This infant's significant hypoglycaemia should be actively, promptly treated with intravenous dextrose, since this specific, correctable metabolic derangement directly, mechanistically explains this infant's own seizure activity and requires urgent, immediate correction

C. This infant should genuinely receive an anticonvulsant medication alone, without any active correction of this significantly low glucose

D. This specific glucose value carries no genuine, established relationship to seizure activity of any kind

E. This infant's own seizure should genuinely be observed for several additional hours before any active, specific intervention

Answer: B. **This infant's significant hypoglycaemia should be actively, promptly treated with intravenous dextrose, since this specific, correctable metabolic derangement directly explains the seizure activity and requires urgent correction.**

This vignette presents significant, symptomatic hypoglycaemia directly producing seizure activity, this specific, connected presentation representing a genuine medical emergency requiring urgent, immediate correction rather than delayed observation or treatment addressing seizure activity alone without correcting this same, underlying cause.

Correct, immediate management directly requires prompt intravenous dextrose administration, this specific intervention directly addressing the underlying metabolic derangement this seizure activity reflects, reinforcing this book's own repeated theme that correctly identifying and treating a specific, underlying cause represents essential, rather than optional, clinical practice.

Treating seizure activity with an anticonvulsant alone, without actively correcting this significant, underlying hypoglycaemia, would provide genuinely limited, incomplete benefit, directly illustrating this book's own repeated theme that correcting a specific finding's own symptom alone, without addressing its own genuine, underlying cause, provides limited, incomplete clinical value.

Why the other options are wrong

A. This seizure activity is directly, mechanistically connected to this infant's own concurrent, significant hypoglycaemia.

C. Active correction of this significant hypoglycaemia, not an anticonvulsant alone, represents the correct, immediate priority.

D. A direct, established, mechanistic relationship exists between this glucose value and seizure activity.

E. Urgent, immediate intervention, not delayed observation, represents the correct, appropriate approach to this specific finding.

Board Alert Significant, symptomatic hypoglycaemia producing seizure activity requires urgent, immediate intravenous dextrose correction, not anticonvulsant treatment or observation alone.

Question 20

A 25-week gestation infant is 4 weeks old and being evaluated for a significant, new heart murmur. The clinical team notes that a previous course of pharmacologic ductal closure was unsuccessful. Which of the following best reflects the correct, current, evidence-based next step in management?

A. No further, active management is genuinely warranted, since a single, unsuccessful pharmacologic course definitively excludes any further, specific treatment option

B. Current management includes active consideration of a further pharmacologic course, continued conservative, expectant management with close monitoring, or surgical ligation, depending on this infant's own specific, connected clinical circumstance, reflecting genuinely current, ongoing evolution in this specific area's own evidence base

C. Surgical ligation represents the only medically acceptable approach in every specific circumstance following an unsuccessful pharmacologic course

D. This infant's own specific, connected clinical circumstance carries no genuine relevance to correctly selecting a further, appropriate management approach

E. This finding requires no further, active clinical attention of any kind following this initial, unsuccessful treatment course

Answer: B. **Current management includes active consideration of a further pharmacologic course, continued conservative management, or surgical ligation, depending on this infant's own specific, connected clinical circumstance, reflecting genuinely current, ongoing evidence evolution.**

This vignette directly tests this book's own established cardiovascular content: management of a haemodynamically significant patent ductus arteriosus has genuinely, considerably evolved, with genuinely current evidence supporting a range of approaches rather than a single, uniform, reflexive intervention following an unsuccessful initial course.

Correct, current practice requires actively weighing this infant's own specific, connected clinical circumstance together, rather than assuming a single approach, whether repeated pharmacologic treatment or immediate, definitive surgical ligation, represents the universally correct, single next step in every specific circumstance.

This reflects this book's own repeated theme that correctly, safely managing a genuinely important, connected cardiovascular finding requires individualised, evidence-based clinical judgment, honestly incorporating genuinely current, still-evolving evidence rather than a single, rigid, historical treatment algorithm applied uniformly.

Why the other options are wrong

A. Further, active management options genuinely remain available following an unsuccessful initial pharmacologic course.

C. A range of approaches, not exclusively surgical ligation, reflects genuinely current, evidence-based management.

D. This infant's own specific circumstance carries direct, essential relevance to selecting the appropriate, further approach.

E. This finding requires continued, active clinical attention and connected management, as detailed in the correct answer.

Board Alert Following unsuccessful pharmacologic ductal closure, current management includes active consideration of a further pharmacologic course, continued conservative management, or surgical ligation, reflecting individualised, evolving evidence.

Question 21

A 26-week gestation infant develops significant abdominal distension, feeding intolerance, and grossly bloody stools on day 12 of life. Abdominal radiography shows pneumatosis intestinalis without pneumoperitoneum. Thrombocytopenia and a rising C-reactive protein are noted. Which of the following best reflects the correct, initial management approach?

A. Immediate surgical exploration is mandatory in this specific circumstance, since pneumatosis intestinalis alone represents an absolute surgical indication

B. Medical management, including bowel rest, broad-spectrum antibiotics, and close, active clinical and laboratory monitoring, represents the correct, initial approach, since pneumoperitoneum, rather than pneumatosis intestinalis alone, represents the sole absolute indication for immediate surgical intervention

C. This infant requires no further, active clinical attention of any kind, since this presentation is entirely self-limited

D. This specific presentation carries no genuine relationship to necrotising enterocolitis of any kind

E. Enteral feeding should genuinely, immediately be advanced despite this specific presentation

Answer: B. Medical management — bowel rest, broad-spectrum antibiotics, and close monitoring — represents the correct, initial approach, since pneumoperitoneum, not pneumatosis intestinalis alone, is the sole absolute surgical indication.

This vignette directly tests this book's own foundational surgical content: pneumoperitoneum, radiological evidence of free intraperitoneal air directly indicating bowel perforation, represents the sole absolute indication for immediate surgical intervention in necrotising enterocolitis.

Pneumatosis intestinalis alone, together with thrombocytopenia and a rising C-reactive protein, represents genuinely important, connected findings requiring active, dynamic clinical monitoring, but not this specific, single, unambiguous surgical indication this book has established throughout.

Correct, initial management therefore appropriately requires medical management — bowel rest, broad-spectrum antibiotics, and close, active, structured monitoring — reflecting this book's own repeated theme that this genuinely uncertain surgical decision-making landscape requires dynamic, individualised assessment short of this single, absolute indication.

Why the other options are wrong

A. Pneumatosis intestinalis alone does not represent an absolute surgical indication; pneumoperitoneum specifically does.

C. This presentation requires active, structured clinical attention, not an assumption of entirely self-limited resolution.

D. This presentation is directly, classically consistent with necrotising enterocolitis, as detailed in the correct answer.

E. Bowel rest, not advancing enteral feeding, represents the correct, initial approach in this specific presentation.

Board Alert Pneumatosis intestinalis alone, without pneumoperitoneum, warrants medical management with bowel rest, antibiotics, and close monitoring — not immediate, mandatory surgical exploration.

Mock Exam 2 — Section B: Organ Systems | Universal Task 4: Management, Treatment and Prevention

Question 22

A term infant born via vacuum-assisted vaginal delivery develops a firm, well-demarcated, non-blanching swelling over the right parietal scalp that does not cross suture lines, noted on day 2 of life. Which of the following best reflects the correct, current understanding of this specific finding?

A. This presentation represents caput succedaneum, a benign, diffuse, superficial swelling crossing suture lines, requiring no further, active evaluation

B. This presentation is more consistent with cephalohaematoma, a subperiosteal haemorrhage that characteristically does not cross suture lines, and while generally self-limited, this finding warrants active, connected monitoring for significant hyperbilirubinaemia as this same collection is gradually reabsorbed

C. This presentation requires immediate, active surgical drainage regardless of clinical stability

D. This specific finding carries no genuine, connected relevance to this infant's own risk of hyperbilirubinaemia

E. This presentation should be managed with immediate, broad-spectrum antibiotic therapy alone

Answer: B. This presentation is more consistent with cephalohaematoma — a subperiosteal haemorrhage that characteristically does not cross suture lines — warranting active monitoring for connected hyperbilirubinaemia as it is gradually reabsorbed.

This vignette directly tests the classic distinction between caput succedaneum and cephalohaematoma: this specific presentation's own well-demarcated borders that do not cross suture lines directly reflect cephalohaematoma's own characteristic, subperiosteal location, genuinely distinct from caput succedaneum's own diffuse, superficial swelling that does cross suture lines.

This same finding is generally self-limited, but directly warrants active, connected monitoring for significant hyperbilirubinaemia, since this same, gradually reabsorbed blood collection directly contributes additional bilirubin load as this same collection is broken down over the subsequent days to weeks.

This reflects this book's own repeated theme that correctly, precisely distinguishing between two, genuinely similar-appearing specific findings directly informs both correct diagnosis and the appropriate, connected clinical monitoring this same finding genuinely requires.

Why the other options are wrong

A. This presentation's specific, well-demarcated borders not crossing suture lines are more consistent with cephalohaematoma.

C. This generally self-limited finding does not require immediate, active surgical drainage regardless of stability.

D. A direct, connected relevance exists between this finding and hyperbilirubinaemia risk, as detailed in the correct answer.

E. This presentation does not require immediate, broad-spectrum antibiotic therapy in the absence of specific, connected infectious concern.

Board Alert Cephalohaematoma, a subperiosteal haemorrhage not crossing suture lines, is generally self-limited but warrants monitoring for connected hyperbilirubinaemia as this collection is gradually reabsorbed.

Question 23

A term infant develops significant respiratory distress and is noted to have absent breath sounds on the left with bowel sounds audible in the left chest, together with significant, associated cardiac and vertebral anomalies on subsequent evaluation. Which of the following best reflects the correct, connected diagnostic consideration this combination of findings should prompt?

A. This infant's combination of findings carries no genuine, connected relationship to any broader, recognised pattern of anomalies

B. This infant's combination of findings should prompt active evaluation for the VACTERL association, given this infant's own confirmed congenital diaphragmatic hernia together with connected cardiac and vertebral anomalies, requiring structured, further evaluation for additional, potentially connected findings

C. This infant's cardiac and vertebral anomalies are entirely coincidental and unrelated to this infant's own confirmed diaphragmatic hernia

D. Congenital diaphragmatic hernia carries no genuine, established relationship to any broader, connected pattern of anomalies

E. This infant requires no further, structured evaluation for any additional, potentially connected anomaly

Answer: B. This combination should prompt active evaluation for the VACTERL association, given confirmed congenital diaphragmatic hernia together with connected cardiac and vertebral anomalies, requiring structured evaluation for additional, potentially connected findings.

This vignette directly tests this book's own established, foundational pattern-recognition principle: a syndrome reflects a single, identified underlying cause, while an association, VACTERL specifically, reflects a genuinely specific, recognised pattern of connected anomalies occurring together at a considerably greater frequency than genuinely expected by chance alone.

This infant's combination of confirmed congenital diaphragmatic hernia together with connected cardiac and vertebral anomalies directly reflects this same, established VACTERL pattern, meaning correctly, completely evaluating this infant requires actively, structurally evaluating for these further, connected anomalies — tracheo-oesophageal, renal, and limb — rather than treating each specific finding as an entirely isolated, unconnected condition.

This reflects this book's own repeated theme that correctly, precisely recognising a genuinely established, connected pattern of anomalies directly informs the appropriate, comprehensive diagnostic evaluation a given infant genuinely requires, extending well beyond this infant's own initially, most apparent presenting finding.

Why the other options are wrong

A. A direct, well-established, connected relationship exists, as detailed in the correct answer, not an absence of relationship.

C. These findings are directly, connectedly related through this established, recognised pattern, not entirely coincidental.

D. Congenital diaphragmatic hernia carries a direct, established relationship to this broader, connected pattern.

E. Active, structured evaluation for additional, connected anomalies is genuinely warranted in this specific presentation.

Board Alert Congenital diaphragmatic hernia together with connected cardiac and vertebral anomalies should prompt active evaluation for the VACTERL association and its further, connected component anomalies.

Mock Exam 2 — Section B: Organ Systems | Universal Task 4: Management, Treatment and Prevention

Question 24

A 27-week gestation infant is 3 weeks old and has been diagnosed with culture-confirmed, late-onset sepsis due to Escherichia coli. The clinical team is reviewing this infant's own overall infection risk profile. Which of the following best reflects a genuinely important, connected consideration regarding this population's own genuine susceptibility to this type of infection?

A. This population's own immune function carries no genuine relationship to infection susceptibility of any kind

B. This population's own genuinely immature immune function, reflecting an extended, ongoing postnatal maturation timeline this book has established throughout, directly helps explain this population's own genuinely elevated, connected infection susceptibility, supporting continued, active vigilance for further, connected infectious complications

C. This population's immune function achieves full, complete maturity immediately following birth, with no genuine, ongoing postnatal development of any kind

D. This infant's own specific infection carries no genuine, connected relevance to this population's own broader immunological status

E. Continued, active vigilance for further, connected infectious complications is genuinely unwarranted following successful treatment

Answer: B. **This population's genuinely immature immune function, reflecting an extended, ongoing postnatal maturation timeline, directly helps explain elevated infection susceptibility, supporting continued, active vigilance for further complications.**

This vignette directly tests this book's own established, extended maturation content: neonatal immune function genuinely, gradually matures over an extended postnatal timeline extending well beyond the immediate neonatal period, this same, extended theme established throughout this book for multiple, distinct organ systems together.

This specific, genuinely incomplete immune competence directly connects to and directly helps explain this population's own genuinely elevated, well-established infection susceptibility, reinforcing this book's repeated, cross-volume demonstration that a specific, foundational physiological maturation timeline directly explains a further, genuinely important, connected clinical vulnerability.

This reflects this book's own repeated theme that correctly, completely understanding this population's own genuine, elevated infection risk requires active, ongoing clinical vigilance extending well beyond a single, successfully treated infectious episode, given this same, underlying immunological immaturity's own genuinely extended, ongoing timeline.

Why the other options are wrong

A. A direct, well-established relationship exists between immune function and infection susceptibility, as detailed in the correct answer.

C. This population's immune function genuinely, gradually matures over an extended timeline, not achieving full maturity immediately at birth.

D. This infant's own specific infection carries direct, connected relevance to this population's own broader immunological status.

E. Continued, active vigilance remains genuinely warranted, given this population's own ongoing, elevated susceptibility.

Board Alert Neonatal immune function genuinely, gradually matures over an extended postnatal timeline, directly helping explain this population's genuinely elevated infection susceptibility and supporting continued, active vigilance.

Question 25

A term infant develops significant respiratory distress within minutes of birth. Auscultation reveals decreased breath sounds on the left with bowel sounds present in the chest. Prenatal imaging had been unremarkable, and this infant's presentation is genuinely delayed relative to the more classic, immediate presentation this book has otherwise emphasised. Which of the following best reflects the correct, honest understanding of this specific clinical circumstance?

A. Congenital diaphragmatic hernia always, exclusively presents during the immediate neonatal period, making this specific, delayed presentation inconsistent with this diagnosis

B. Genuinely current, specific case series evidence has directly documented late-presenting congenital diaphragmatic hernia, this specific, genuinely rare presentation frequently, genuinely leading to misdiagnosis given the genuine absence of the classic, immediate respiratory distress this book has otherwise established as this condition's own characteristic presentation

C. This infant's presentation carries no genuine relationship to congenital diaphragmatic hernia of any kind, given prior, unremarkable prenatal imaging

D. This specific, later presentation carries an identical, equally straightforward diagnosis to the classic, immediate neonatal presentation

E. Prenatal imaging always, definitively excludes this specific diagnosis when genuinely unremarkable

Answer: B. Genuinely current case series evidence documents late-presenting congenital diaphragmatic hernia, this genuinely rare presentation frequently leading to misdiagnosis given the genuine absence of the classic, immediate respiratory distress this book otherwise emphasises.

This vignette directly tests this book's own honest, genuinely current acknowledgement of an important exception to the classic presentation: genuinely current, specific case series evidence has directly documented late-presenting congenital diaphragmatic hernia, occurring genuinely beyond the immediate neonatal period.

This specific, genuinely rare presentation frequently, genuinely leads to misdiagnosis given the genuine, complete absence of the classic, immediate respiratory distress this book's earlier content has established as this condition's own characteristic, defining presentation, directly explaining why prior, unremarkable prenatal imaging does not entirely, definitively exclude this specific diagnosis.

This reflects this book's own repeated theme that correctly, completely understanding a specific structural anomaly requires actively considering genuine, current exceptions to even a genuinely well-established, classically taught presentation, rather than assuming every affected infant genuinely conforms to a single, familiar clinical picture.

Why the other options are wrong

A. A genuine, later presentation is genuinely possible, as detailed in the correct answer, not exclusively immediate presentation.

C. This presentation carries direct, genuine relevance to this diagnosis, despite prior, unremarkable prenatal imaging.

D. This later presentation carries a genuinely more difficult, not equally straightforward, diagnosis given absent classic findings.

E. Prior, unremarkable prenatal imaging does not entirely, definitively exclude this specific diagnosis, as detailed in the correct answer.

Board Alert Genuinely current case series document late-presenting congenital diaphragmatic hernia, frequently leading to misdiagnosis given the absence of classic, immediate respiratory distress and despite prior, unremarkable prenatal imaging.

Question 26

A 30-week gestation infant is 5 days old and has developed significant, progressive direct hyperbilirubinaemia while receiving full parenteral nutrition support with minimal enteral intake. Which of the following represents the most appropriate, active management consideration?

A. No specific, active management consideration exists for this specific finding of any kind

B. Active consideration of advancing enteral feeds where genuinely, clinically possible represents a genuinely important, established strategy for both preventing and managing parenteral nutrition-associated cholestasis, this specific finding's own most likely, connected explanation

C. This finding should be managed exclusively with continued, unchanged parenteral nutrition, without any genuine, active reconsideration of feeding strategy

D. This specific finding carries no genuine, connected relationship to this infant's own duration or composition of nutritional support

E. This finding requires no further, active evaluation or connected management of any kind

Answer: B. **Active consideration of advancing enteral feeds where genuinely possible represents an established strategy for both preventing and managing parenteral nutrition-associated cholestasis, this finding's most likely, connected explanation.**

This vignette directly tests this book's own established nutrition content: a predominantly direct hyperbilirubinaemia occurring in the setting of prolonged parenteral nutrition with minimal enteral intake is most consistent with parenteral nutrition-associated cholestasis, a genuinely important, recognised complication particularly relevant in the preterm population.
This same finding directly, practically supports active consideration of advancing enteral feeds where genuinely, clinically possible, since this same, active transition toward enteral nutrition represents a genuinely important, established strategy for both preventing and managing this specific, connected complication.

This reflects this book's own repeated theme that correctly, actively managing a specific, connected nutritional complication requires active reconsideration of this infant's own overall feeding strategy, rather than passive continuation of an unchanged approach that may itself be directly contributing to this same, ongoing complication.

Why the other options are wrong

A. A genuine, active management consideration exists, as detailed in the correct answer, not an absence of consideration.

C. Active reconsideration of feeding strategy, not continued, unchanged parenteral nutrition alone, represents the correct approach.

D. A direct, established relationship exists between nutritional support duration and this specific complication.

E. Active evaluation and connected management are genuinely warranted for this specific finding.

Board Alert A predominantly direct hyperbilirubinaemia during prolonged parenteral nutrition is most consistent with parenteral nutrition-associated cholestasis, supporting active consideration of advancing enteral feeds where possible.

Mock Exam 2 — Section B: Organ Systems | Universal Task 3: Diagnosis, Testing and Monitoring

Question 27

A 25-week gestation infant is 6 weeks old and undergoing routine ophthalmologic screening for retinopathy of prematurity. The examining ophthalmologist identifies findings meeting current, established treatment criteria. Which of the following best reflects the correct, immediate next step?

A. No specific, active treatment is genuinely warranted at this stage, regardless of this specific ophthalmologic finding

B. Prompt, timely treatment should be initiated according to current, established criteria, since correctly, actively monitoring this genuinely dynamic condition directly determines the correct, timely moment for treatment intervention once genuine progression meeting these criteria has actually occurred

C. This specific finding should genuinely be reassessed in 3 further months before any active treatment consideration

D. This infant's own gestational age carries no genuine relevance to correctly determining appropriate treatment timing

E. This specific condition never, genuinely warrants active treatment regardless of examination findings

Answer: B. Prompt, timely treatment should be initiated according to current, established criteria, since active, structured surveillance exists precisely to determine the correct, timely moment for intervention once genuine progression occurs.

This vignette directly tests this book's own established ophthalmology content: structured, serial ophthalmologic examinations continue on an appropriate, individualised schedule precisely because retinopathy of prematurity can genuinely progress, and serial monitoring directly informs the correct, timely decision regarding treatment when genuinely indicated.

Once this same, structured surveillance identifies findings genuinely meeting current, established treatment criteria, prompt, timely treatment represents the correct, appropriate next step, reflecting this book's own repeated theme that correctly, safely managing this genuinely dynamic condition requires acting decisively once active monitoring has identified this same, genuine, defined threshold.

This reflects this book's own repeated theme that a genuinely structured, ongoing surveillance programme exists specifically to enable timely, appropriate intervention, rather than surveillance alone without eventual, decisive action once genuine, established criteria are actually met.

Why the other options are wrong

A. Active treatment is genuinely warranted once established criteria are met, as detailed in the correct answer.

C. Prompt, timely treatment, not further, extended delay, represents the correct approach once criteria are genuinely met.

D. This infant's own gestational age carries direct, genuine relevance to this condition's own broader risk and management context.

E. This condition genuinely warrants active treatment once specific, established criteria are met, as detailed in the correct answer.

Board Alert Once structured, serial ophthalmologic surveillance identifies findings meeting current, established treatment criteria for retinopathy of prematurity, prompt, timely treatment represents the correct, appropriate next step.

Question 28

A 24-week gestation infant is receiving structured, longer-term follow-up after a course of ECMO support for severe respiratory failure related to congenital diaphragmatic hernia. Which of the following best reflects the correct, comprehensive understanding of this infant's own ongoing care needs?

A. This infant's own clinical needs conclude entirely once the acute period of ECMO support has ended, with no genuine, further, structured follow-up required

B. This infant's own care requires structured, longer-term neurodevelopmental follow-up, directly connecting to this book's own genuinely current ECMO follow-up guideline content, extending clinical attention well beyond the acute period of support itself given this population's own genuinely elevated, connected vulnerability

C. ECMO support carries no genuine, connected relationship to this infant's own longer-term neurodevelopmental outcome of any kind

D. This infant's own underlying congenital diaphragmatic hernia carries no genuine relevance to this infant's own ongoing, structured follow-up needs

E. This infant requires no further, active coordination between neonatology and any other, connected clinical discipline

Answer: B. **This infant's care requires structured, longer-term neurodevelopmental follow-up, directly connecting to this book's genuinely current ECMO follow-up guideline content, extending attention well beyond the acute period given this population's genuinely elevated, connected vulnerability.**

This vignette directly tests this book's own genuinely current ECMO follow-up content: genuinely current, specific clinical guidelines directly address structured, longer-term follow-up after neonatal ECMO, this genuinely current guideline directly connecting to this book's own extensive neurodevelopmental follow-up content established throughout its earlier volumes.

This means correctly, completely managing an infant who has genuinely received this technology requires actively, deliberately extending clinical attention well beyond the immediate, acute period of support itself, into this infant's own considerably longer-term, connected developmental trajectory.

This reflects this book's own repeated, closing theme that a genuinely important acute intervention established throughout this book directly, connectedly extends into this infant's own considerably longer-term, connected clinical course, requiring the same, structured, coordinated, multidisciplinary attention this book has established repeatedly throughout its entire span.

Why the other options are wrong

A. Structured, longer-term follow-up remains genuinely required, not concluding entirely once acute support has ended.

C. A direct, established, connected relationship exists between ECMO support and longer-term outcome, as detailed in the correct answer.

D. This infant's own underlying diagnosis carries direct, genuine relevance to this infant's own ongoing follow-up needs.

E. This infant genuinely requires coordinated, multidisciplinary involvement, not an absence of this coordination.

Board Alert Genuinely current ECMO follow-up guidelines directly connect to this book's extensive neurodevelopmental follow-up content, requiring structured, longer-term attention well beyond the acute period of support.

Question 29

A term infant develops significant respiratory distress, is noted to have a small, receding chin along with a cleft palate, and demonstrates significant, intermittent airway obstruction particularly when positioned supine. Which of the following best reflects the correct, connected diagnostic consideration and immediate management approach?

A. This combination of findings carries no genuine, connected relationship to any broader, recognised pattern of anomalies

B. This presentation is highly consistent with Pierre Robin sequence, in which micrognathia directly leads to glossoptosis and connected airway obstruction, meaning correctly, immediately positioning this infant prone, rather than supine, often provides genuine, immediate improvement while further, definitive management is considered

C. This infant should genuinely, always be positioned supine regardless of this specific, connected presentation

D. Cleft palate in this specific context carries no genuine, connected relevance to this infant's own airway obstruction

E. This presentation requires no further, active management of any kind beyond simple, passive observation

Answer: B. This presentation is highly consistent with Pierre Robin sequence, in which micrognathia directly leads to glossoptosis and connected airway obstruction — prone positioning often provides immediate improvement while further management is considered.

This vignette presents the classic, connected triad of Pierre Robin sequence: micrognathia (a small, receding chin), glossoptosis (posteriorly displaced tongue), and cleft palate together, this specific, connected sequence directly explaining this infant's own significant, positional airway obstruction.

This connected mechanism directly explains why prone positioning often provides genuine, immediate improvement: this specific position directly allows the tongue to fall forward, away from the posterior pharyngeal wall, directly relieving this same, connected obstruction that supine positioning otherwise, directly worsens.

This reflects this book's own repeated theme that correctly, precisely understanding a specific, connected anatomical sequence directly informs an immediate, practical, bedside management strategy, while further, definitive management, potentially including specific surgical intervention, is actively considered.

Why the other options are wrong

A. A direct, well-established, connected relationship exists between these findings and this specific, recognised sequence.

C. Prone, not supine, positioning often provides genuine, immediate improvement in this specific presentation.

D. This specific finding carries direct, connected relevance to this infant's own broader presentation, as detailed in the correct answer.

E. Active management, including positioning and further, definitive consideration, is genuinely warranted for this presentation.

Board Alert Pierre Robin sequence: micrognathia leads to glossoptosis and connected airway obstruction. Prone positioning often provides immediate improvement while further, definitive management is considered.

Question 30

A 28-week gestation infant is 3 weeks old and has a confirmed, grade III intraventricular haemorrhage. The family asks the clinical team about this infant's own eventual, longer-term outcome. Which of the following best reflects the correct, honest, and complete response to this specific family question?

A. This infant's own longer-term outcome can be predicted with entirely complete, absolute certainty at this specific, early point in this infant's own clinical course

B. Honest, complete counselling requires acknowledging genuine, remaining uncertainty regarding this infant's own specific, eventual outcome, while actively committing to the same structured, longer-term neurodevelopmental follow-up this book has established as essential for correctly, safely monitoring this same, genuine trajectory over time

C. This specific family question deserves no genuine, substantive response of any kind

D. This infant's own current, confirmed finding carries no genuine relevance to this infant's own longer-term outcome

E. Structured, longer-term follow-up carries no genuine relevance to correctly addressing this specific family question

Answer: B. **Honest, complete counselling requires acknowledging genuine, remaining uncertainty regarding eventual outcome, while committing to the same structured, longer-term follow-up this book establishes as essential for monitoring this trajectory over time.**

This vignette directly tests this book's own repeated, honest communication principle applied to a genuinely important, common family question following a significant neurological finding: correctly, compassionately responding requires honestly acknowledging genuine, remaining uncertainty regarding this infant's own specific, eventual outcome.

This same, honest response directly connects to this book's own established neurology content: significant grade III intraventricular haemorrhage carries genuine, established relevance to this infant's own longer-term neurodevelopmental outcome, supporting the same structured, longer-term follow-up this book has established throughout as essential for this population.

This reflects this book's own repeated theme that honest, complete communication with a family requires actively acknowledging genuine uncertainty while still providing this same family with a clear, concrete, and genuinely reassuring plan for ongoing, structured, and connected clinical attention over this infant's own entire, connected developmental journey.

Why the other options are wrong

A. Genuine, remaining uncertainty exists at this early stage, as detailed in the correct answer, not entirely complete certainty.

C. This specific family question deserves a genuine, substantive, honest response, as detailed in the correct answer.

D. This infant's own current finding carries direct, genuine relevance to this infant's own longer-term outcome.

E. This follow-up carries direct, genuine relevance to addressing this specific family question, as detailed in the correct answer.

Board Alert Honest counselling following a significant intraventricular haemorrhage acknowledges genuine, remaining uncertainty regarding eventual outcome while committing to structured, longer-term follow-up.

Question 31

A term infant develops significant, progressive jaundice on day 2 of life. Total bilirubin is markedly elevated. A maternal history reveals significant, previously diagnosed glucose-6-phosphate dehydrogenase deficiency risk given family ancestry, though this infant's own specific status is not yet known. Which of the following best reflects the correct, immediate diagnostic consideration?

A. This family history carries no genuine relevance to correctly evaluating this infant's own significant jaundice

B. Active testing for glucose-6-phosphate dehydrogenase deficiency should genuinely be considered, since this specific, X-linked enzymatic deficiency can directly produce significant, potentially severe hemolysis and hyperbilirubinaemia, particularly relevant given this infant's own specific, connected family history and ancestry

C. This presentation should be managed exclusively as physiologic jaundice, without any further, specific diagnostic evaluation

D. This specific enzymatic deficiency carries no genuine, established relationship to significant hyperbilirubinaemia of any kind

E. This infant's own significant jaundice requires no further, active clinical attention given this presentation's timing

Answer: B. Active testing for glucose-6-phosphate dehydrogenase deficiency should be considered, since this X-linked enzymatic deficiency can directly produce significant, potentially severe hemolysis and hyperbilirubinaemia, particularly relevant given this infant's connected family history and ancestry.

This vignette directly tests active, connected consideration of glucose-6-phosphate dehydrogenase deficiency, a specific, X-linked enzymatic deficiency directly capable of producing significant, potentially severe hemolysis and correspondingly significant hyperbilirubinaemia, particularly relevant given specific, connected family history and ancestry.

This infant's own significant, day-2 jaundice, occurring earlier and more significantly than typical, physiologic jaundice, together with this specific, connected family history, directly supports active, prompt diagnostic testing rather than reflexive attribution to physiologic jaundice alone.

This reflects this book's own repeated theme that correctly, actively identifying a specific, underlying, potentially treatable cause of significant hyperbilirubinaemia directly requires active consideration of connected, relevant family history, rather than assuming every case of significant jaundice reflects an identical, benign, physiologic process.

Why the other options are wrong

A. This family history carries direct, genuine relevance to correctly evaluating this infant, as detailed in the correct answer.

C. This presentation, given its timing and connected family history, warrants active, specific diagnostic evaluation.

D. A direct, established relationship exists between this deficiency and significant hyperbilirubinaemia, as detailed in the correct answer.

E. This finding warrants active, prompt clinical attention, not an absence of further consideration.

Board Alert Glucose-6-phosphate dehydrogenase deficiency, an X-linked enzymatic deficiency, can produce significant hemolysis and hyperbilirubinaemia — active testing should be considered given connected family history and ancestry.

Question 32

A 26-week gestation infant is 2 weeks old and has developed significant, progressive abdominal distension. Abdominal radiography demonstrates a specific pattern suggesting spontaneous intestinal perforation, genuinely distinct from classic necrotising enterocolitis, in an infant who has not yet been significantly, enterally fed. Which of the following best reflects a genuinely important, connected risk factor for this specific, distinct condition?

A. This specific condition carries an identical underlying mechanism and risk factor profile to classic necrotising enterocolitis

B. Early postnatal corticosteroid exposure and concurrent indomethacin administration have each been associated with spontaneous intestinal perforation, a specific condition genuinely distinct from classic necrotising enterocolitis in its own underlying mechanism, timing, and connected risk factor profile

C. This specific condition carries no genuine, established, connected risk factor of any kind

D. Enteral feeding status carries no genuine relevance to distinguishing this specific condition from classic necrotising enterocolitis

E. This specific condition requires an identical management approach to classic necrotising enterocolitis in every specific circumstance

Answer: B. **Early postnatal corticosteroid exposure and concurrent indomethacin administration have each been associated with spontaneous intestinal perforation, a condition genuinely distinct from classic necrotising enterocolitis in mechanism, timing, and risk factor profile.**

This vignette directly tests an important, genuinely distinct condition from classic necrotising enterocolitis: spontaneous intestinal perforation typically occurs earlier, often in infants not yet significantly enterally fed, and carries a genuinely different, specific underlying mechanism and connected risk factor profile.

Early postnatal corticosteroid exposure and concurrent indomethacin administration have each been specifically associated with this distinct condition, directly connecting to this book's own established pharmacology content regarding indomethacin's own genuine, established connected risks.

This reflects this book's own repeated theme that correctly, precisely distinguishing between two, genuinely similar-appearing but mechanistically distinct conditions directly informs both correct diagnosis and appropriate, targeted management, rather than assuming an identical approach applies uniformly across genuinely different, underlying pathophysiology.

Why the other options are wrong

A. This condition carries a genuinely distinct, not identical, underlying mechanism and risk factor profile.

C. Specific, established, connected risk factors exist, as detailed in the correct answer, not an absence of risk factors.

D. Enteral feeding status and timing carry direct, distinguishing relevance between these two, genuinely distinct conditions.

E. This condition's own genuinely distinct mechanism may inform a genuinely different, specific management approach.

Board Alert Spontaneous intestinal perforation is genuinely distinct from classic necrotising enterocolitis in mechanism and timing; early postnatal corticosteroids and concurrent indomethacin are each associated risk factors.

Question 33

A term infant develops significant respiratory distress, and auscultation reveals significantly decreased breath sounds bilaterally with a specific, 'washing machine' murmur noted on cardiac examination. Echocardiography confirms truncus arteriosus. Which of the following best explains the connected, underlying physiologic consequence of this specific structural cardiac lesion?

A. This specific lesion carries no genuine, connected physiologic consequence of any kind

B. This specific lesion, in which a single, common arterial trunk arises from the heart supplying both systemic and pulmonary circulation together, directly produces significant mixing of oxygenated and deoxygenated blood, with connected pulmonary overcirculation as pulmonary vascular resistance normally falls following birth

C. This specific lesion produces complete, physiologic separation between systemic and pulmonary circulation, identical to a structurally normal heart

D. Pulmonary vascular resistance carries no genuine, connected relevance to this specific lesion's own physiologic consequence

E. This specific murmur carries no genuine, diagnostic significance in this specific clinical context

Answer: B. **Truncus arteriosus produces significant mixing of oxygenated and deoxygenated blood through a single, common arterial trunk, with connected pulmonary overcirculation as pulmonary vascular resistance normally falls following birth.**

This vignette presents truncus arteriosus, in which a single, common arterial trunk arises from the heart and supplies both the systemic and pulmonary circulation together, directly producing significant, connected mixing of oxygenated and deoxygenated blood at this single, shared vascular origin.

This same, connected structural lesion directly produces progressive pulmonary overcirculation as pulmonary vascular resistance normally, physiologically falls following birth, this same, expected postnatal transition this book has established at length throughout its own physiology content directly worsening, rather than improving, this infant's own connected haemodynamic status in this specific structural circumstance.

This reflects this book's own repeated theme that a specific, structural cardiac lesion's own genuine, connected physiologic consequence frequently depends directly on this same infant's own broader, connected physiological transition, rather than this same lesion's own structural description alone providing an entirely complete clinical picture.

Why the other options are wrong

A. A direct, significant, connected physiologic consequence exists, as detailed in the correct answer, not an absence of consequence.

C. This lesion produces significant mixing, not complete, physiologic separation identical to a structurally normal heart.

D. A direct, connected relevance exists between pulmonary vascular resistance and this lesion's own consequence.

E. This specific murmur carries direct, diagnostic significance in this specific clinical context.

> **Board Alert** Truncus arteriosus produces significant mixing of oxygenated and deoxygenated blood, with connected pulmonary overcirculation worsening as pulmonary vascular resistance normally falls following birth.

Question 34

A 29-week gestation infant is 10 days old and has developed significant hyponatraemia while receiving standard maintenance parenteral fluids. Urine output remains adequate. Which of the following represents an important, connected consideration in correctly evaluating this specific finding?

A. This finding carries no genuine, connected relationship to this infant's own gestational age or renal maturation of any kind

B. This infant's own genuinely immature renal function, directly connecting to the extended, ongoing glomerular filtration rate maturation content this book establishes throughout, carries genuine, connected relevance to correctly interpreting this infant's own significant hyponatraemia and appropriately adjusting connected fluid and electrolyte management

C. This finding requires no further, active evaluation or connected management of any kind

D. This infant's own current postnatal age carries no genuine relevance to correctly interpreting this specific finding

E. Standard, unmodified adult electrolyte management principles apply identically and directly to this specific infant

> **Answer: B. This infant's own genuinely immature renal function, directly connecting to the extended glomerular filtration rate maturation content this book establishes, carries genuine relevance to correctly interpreting this hyponatraemia and adjusting fluid and electrolyte management.**
>
> This vignette directly tests this book's own established content regarding extended, ongoing renal maturation: glomerular filtration rate genuinely, gradually matures over the first several weeks and months following birth, meaning correctly interpreting a given infant's own renal function at any specific point requires actively considering this same infant's own specific postnatal, as well as gestational, age.
>
> This same, genuinely immature renal function directly carries connected

relevance to this infant's own capacity for sodium handling and free water excretion, directly informing correctly, safely interpreting this specific finding and appropriately, individually adjusting this infant's own connected fluid and electrolyte management.

This reflects this book's own repeated theme that correctly, safely managing fluid and electrolyte status in this population requires active, individualised consideration of this infant's own specific, developmentally distinctive renal physiology, rather than applying standard, unmodified adult or even term-infant management principles directly.

Why the other options are wrong

A. A direct, established relationship exists between this finding and renal maturation, as detailed in the correct answer.

C. Active evaluation and connected management are genuinely warranted for this specific finding.

D. This infant's own postnatal age carries direct, genuine relevance to correctly interpreting this specific finding.

E. Individually adjusted, developmentally aware management, not standard adult principles, applies to this specific infant.

Board Alert Genuinely immature renal function, connecting to extended glomerular filtration rate maturation, carries genuine relevance to correctly interpreting hyponatraemia and adjusting fluid and electrolyte management in this population.

Question 35

A term infant develops significant respiratory distress and is noted to have significant micrognathia, low-set ears, and bilateral talipes. Growth parameters are significantly below expected for gestational age. Genetic testing confirms trisomy 18. Which of the following best reflects the correct, honest, and complete counselling this infant's family requires?

A. This family should be provided with a single, generic prognosis identical to that given for trisomy 21

B. This family deserves honest, complete counselling acknowledging this specific diagnosis's own considerably more severe, connected pattern of significant major congenital anomalies and correspondingly more limited overall prognosis compared with trisomy 21, together with the full, complete spectrum of reasonable care options and this family's own genuine, active decision-making authority throughout

C. This specific diagnosis carries an identical prognosis and management approach to trisomy 21 in every specific circumstance

D. This family's own genuine values and preferences carry no genuine relevance to this specific counselling conversation

E. This specific diagnosis requires no further, active or honest discussion of any kind with this family

Answer: B. **This family deserves honest counselling acknowledging trisomy 18's own considerably more severe, connected pattern of anomalies and correspondingly more limited prognosis compared with trisomy 21, together with the full spectrum of options and this family's own genuine decision-making authority.**

This vignette directly tests this book's own established genetics and ethics content together: trisomy 18, genuinely distinct from the more familiar trisomy 21, is directly, characteristically associated with a genuinely broader, considerably more severe pattern of significant major congenital anomalies and a correspondingly, genuinely more limited overall prognosis.

Correctly, precisely distinguishing this genuinely more severe trisomy from trisomy 21 directly informs appropriate, honest antenatal and postnatal family counselling, reinforcing this book's own repeated theme that correctly identifying the specific chromosomal abnormality genuinely present directly determines the appropriate, honest prognostic information a given family genuinely deserves.

This same, honest counselling directly requires the full, complete spectrum of reasonable care options and this family's own genuine, active decision-making authority throughout, precisely the same, connected shared decision-making principle this book has established repeatedly throughout its own ethics content for every genuinely difficult, high-stakes clinical circumstance.

Why the other options are wrong

A. This diagnosis carries a genuinely different, more limited prognosis than trisomy 21, requiring diagnosis-specific counselling.

C. This diagnosis carries a genuinely different, more severe prognosis and connected management approach than trisomy 21.

D. This family's own genuine values carry direct, essential relevance to this counselling conversation.

E. This diagnosis warrants active, honest, and complete discussion with this family, as detailed in the correct answer.

Board Alert Trisomy 18 carries a considerably more severe, connected pattern of anomalies and more limited prognosis than trisomy 21, requiring honest, diagnosis-specific counselling alongside the full spectrum of options.

Question 36

A 25-week gestation infant is 8 weeks old and remains on mechanical ventilation. The clinical team is discussing correctly balancing continuous heparin anticoagulation should this infant require ECMO, against the genuine risk of significant circuit thrombosis. Which of the following best reflects the correct, complete understanding of this specific clinical challenge?

A. This specific balancing challenge carries no genuine, meaningful relevance to correctly, safely managing this chapter's own central technology

B. Correctly, safely balancing continuous heparin anticoagulation against significant circuit thrombosis risk represents a genuinely important, ongoing clinical challenge, since genuinely insufficient anticoagulation risks significant, potentially catastrophic circuit thrombosis, while genuinely excessive anticoagulation directly compounds this population's own already elevated, established bleeding vulnerability

C. Genuinely excessive anticoagulation carries no genuine, compounding relationship to bleeding risk of any kind

D. Circuit thrombosis carries no genuine, meaningful relevance to correctly, safely managing this specific technology

E. This specific challenge requires no genuine, active, continuous, individually titrated balance of any kind

Answer: B. Correctly balancing continuous anticoagulation against significant circuit thrombosis risk represents an important, ongoing challenge, since insufficient anticoagulation

risks catastrophic thrombosis, while excessive anticoagulation compounds this population's already elevated bleeding vulnerability.

This vignette directly tests this book's own established ECMO content: correctly, safely balancing continuous heparin anticoagulation against the equally genuine risk of significant circuit thrombosis represents a genuinely important, ongoing clinical challenge directly extending this book's own established, significant bleeding risk content.

Genuinely insufficient anticoagulation risks significant, potentially catastrophic circuit thrombosis, directly compromising this same technology's own genuine, ongoing function, while genuinely excessive anticoagulation, by contrast, directly compounds this same population's own already elevated, established bleeding vulnerability.

This reflects this book's own repeated theme that correctly, safely applying this chapter's own central technology requires active, continuous, individually titrated balance between these two, genuinely opposing risks, rather than pursuing a single, specific goal without regard to its own connected, opposing risk.

Why the other options are wrong

A. This specific challenge carries direct, essential relevance to safely managing this technology, as detailed in the correct answer.

C. A direct, compounding relationship exists between excessive anticoagulation and bleeding risk, as detailed in the correct answer.

D. This specific risk carries direct, essential relevance to safely managing this technology, as detailed in the correct answer.

E. This specific challenge genuinely requires this same, active, individually titrated balance, as detailed in the correct answer.

Board Alert Correctly balancing continuous heparin anticoagulation against circuit thrombosis risk represents an important, ongoing ECMO challenge, requiring active, continuous, individually titrated balance between these two opposing risks.

Mock Exam 2 — Section B: Organ Systems | Universal Task 3: Diagnosis, Testing and Monitoring

Question 37

A term infant develops significant lethargy, poor feeding, and a bulging fontanelle on day 6 of life. Cerebrospinal fluid analysis confirms significant pleocytosis with elevated protein and low glucose. Blood and cerebrospinal fluid cultures both grow group B Streptococcus. Which of the following best reflects the correct, complete understanding of this infant's own overall condition and its own required management?

A. This infant's confirmed bacteraemia is entirely unrelated to this infant's own confirmed, connected central nervous system findings

B. This infant has confirmed group B Streptococcus meningitis, and correct, complete management requires an extended, specific duration of appropriate intravenous antibiotic therapy directly reflecting this same, confirmed central nervous system involvement, together with active, structured monitoring for connected complications including hydrocephalus and significant hearing loss

C. This infant's cerebrospinal fluid findings carry no genuine, established relationship to this infant's own confirmed bacteraemia

D. This infant requires an identical, standard duration of antibiotic therapy to uncomplicated bacteraemia alone, without any genuine, extended treatment course

E. This infant requires no further, active or structured, connected monitoring following completion of antibiotic therapy

Answer: B. **This infant has confirmed group B Streptococcus meningitis, requiring an extended, specific duration of appropriate antibiotics reflecting confirmed CNS involvement, together with active, structured monitoring for connected complications including hydrocephalus and hearing loss.**

This vignette presents confirmed, culture-positive group B Streptococcus meningitis, this infant's own significant lethargy, poor feeding, bulging fontanelle, and confirmed, connected cerebrospinal fluid findings together directly reflecting genuine, significant central nervous system infection rather than uncomplicated bacteraemia alone.

Correct, complete management directly requires an extended, specific duration of appropriate intravenous antibiotic therapy, genuinely longer than uncomplicated bacteraemia alone would require, this extended duration directly reflecting the genuine, confirmed central nervous system involvement this infant's own cerebrospinal fluid findings confirm.

This same, confirmed diagnosis directly requires active, structured, connected monitoring for significant, established complications, including hydrocephalus and significant hearing loss, reflecting this book's own repeated theme that a confirmed, significant infectious diagnosis frequently carries genuine, connected relevance extending well beyond this infant's own immediate, acute treatment course alone.

Why the other options are wrong

A. This infant's confirmed bacteraemia is directly, mechanistically connected to this infant's own confirmed CNS findings.

C. A direct, established relationship exists between these cerebrospinal fluid findings and this infant's confirmed bacteraemia.

D. This infant requires a genuinely extended, not identical or standard, duration of therapy given confirmed CNS involvement.

E. Active, structured, connected monitoring for complications is genuinely warranted following this confirmed diagnosis.

Board Alert Confirmed group B Streptococcus meningitis requires an extended duration of appropriate antibiotics reflecting confirmed CNS involvement, together with structured monitoring for connected complications including hydrocephalus and hearing loss.

Question 38

A 27-week gestation infant is 4 weeks old and has developed significant metabolic bone disease of prematurity with a markedly elevated alkaline phosphatase and radiographic evidence of significant osteopenia. Which of the following best reflects the correct, connected understanding of this infant's own underlying risk and appropriate management?

A. This finding carries no genuine, connected relationship to this infant's own nutritional support of any kind

B. This population's own genuinely elevated calcium and phosphorus requirements, directly connecting to this book's established human milk fortification content, directly explain this infant's own genuine, elevated risk for this specific condition, supporting active attention to correctly, adequately meeting these same, elevated mineral requirements

C. This finding requires no further, active nutritional or connected management consideration of any kind

D. This infant's own specific gestational age carries no genuine relevance to this infant's own risk for this specific condition

E. Alkaline phosphatase carries no genuine, established relationship to bone mineralisation of any kind

Answer: B. **This population's genuinely elevated calcium and phosphorus requirements, connecting to this book's human milk fortification content, directly explain elevated risk for this condition, supporting active attention to meeting these elevated mineral requirements.**

This vignette directly tests this book's own established nutrition content: the preterm infant's own genuinely elevated nutritional requirements, particularly for calcium and phosphorus, directly connect to this same population's own genuine, elevated risk of metabolic bone disease of prematurity.

This same, connected risk directly reinforces this book's own established human milk fortification content, since unfortified human milk alone typically does not provide sufficient quantities of calcium and phosphorus to meet this population's own elevated requirements, directly supporting active attention to correctly, adequately meeting these same, elevated mineral requirements through appropriate fortification.

This reflects this book's own repeated theme that correctly, individually tailoring nutritional support to this population's own genuinely distinctive requirements directly supports not only overall growth, but this same population's own genuine, connected bone health, requiring active, ongoing nutritional attention throughout this infant's own hospitalisation.

Why the other options are wrong

A. A direct, established relationship exists between this finding and nutritional support, as detailed in the correct answer.

C. Active nutritional and connected management consideration is genuinely warranted for this specific finding.

D. This infant's own gestational age carries direct, genuine relevance to this infant's own risk for this specific condition.

E. A direct, established relationship exists between this marker and bone mineralisation, as detailed in the correct answer.

Board Alert This population's genuinely elevated calcium and phosphorus requirements, connecting to human milk fortification content, directly explain elevated risk for metabolic bone disease of prematurity.

Question 39

A genuinely current, specific quality improvement initiative at a Level 3 NICU targeted improving procedural pain management practices. Baseline data showed fewer than 30 per cent of neonates receiving appropriate pain management interventions for a common, minor procedure. Which of the following best reflects the correct, structured methodology this initiative would most appropriately follow?

A. Immediate, broad, systemwide implementation of a new protocol without any genuine, structured aim or preceding, small-scale trial

B. Formulating a specific, measurable, actionable, realistic, and timely aim — for example, increasing this specific intervention rate from below 30 per cent toward a specific, targeted goal above 50 per cent within a defined period — then applying the Plan-Do-Study-Act cycle beginning with a small-scale trial

C. This specific improvement opportunity requires no genuine, structured methodology of any kind

D. Process measures and outcome measures should genuinely be treated as an identical, interchangeable category throughout this initiative

E. This specific initiative requires no genuine, ongoing measurement or connected evaluation of any kind

Answer: B. **The correct approach formulates a specific SMART aim — for example, increasing intervention rates from below 30 per cent toward a specific, targeted goal above 50 per cent — then applies the Plan-Do-Study-Act cycle beginning with a small-scale trial.**

This vignette directly tests this book's own genuinely current care systems and quality improvement content: a genuinely current quality improvement initiative directly employed the Plan-Do-Study-Act methodology to address procedural pain management, genuinely, measurably increasing the proportion of neonates receiving pain management interventions from a baseline below 30 per cent toward a specific, targeted goal above 50 per cent.

This same, structured approach directly requires formulating a specific, measurable, actionable, realistic, and timely aim before this same initiative's own subsequent implementation actually begins, this same, structured aim directly informing the specific planning phase this methodology genuinely requires.

This reflects this book's own repeated theme that correctly, effectively structuring a given quality improvement initiative requires structured, precisely defined methodology at every genuine stage, beginning with this same initiative's own specific, quantifiable aim, then proceeding through small-scale trial before broader, systemwide implementation.

Why the other options are wrong

A. A structured aim and small-scale trial, not immediate, broad implementation, represents the correct, structured methodology.

C. This specific opportunity benefits from structured, established methodology, as detailed in the correct answer.

D. These represent genuinely distinct, complementary measurement categories, not an identical, interchangeable category.

E. Genuine, ongoing measurement and evaluation are essential components of this specific methodology.

Board Alert A genuinely current pain management QI initiative used the Plan-Do-Study-Act cycle with a specific SMART aim, increasing intervention rates from below 30 per cent toward a targeted goal above 50 per cent.

Question 40

A genuinely current, specific randomised controlled trial reports its own primary outcome result with a 95 per cent confidence interval that is genuinely wide, spanning from a small, clinically negligible benefit to a genuinely substantial, clinically important benefit. Which of the following best reflects the correct, complete interpretation of this specific finding?

A. This wide confidence interval carries no genuine, meaningful relevance to correctly interpreting this trial's own reported result

B. This genuinely wide confidence interval directly reflects genuine, limited precision in this trial's own specific estimate of the true, actual effect, meaning correctly, completely evaluating this trial's own genuine result requires actively considering this same interval's own genuine width, alongside this study's own reported p-value alone, rather than either statistic considered in complete isolation

C. A genuinely wide confidence interval carries an identical, equally precise meaning to a genuinely narrow confidence interval

D. This specific interval's own reported width has no genuine relationship to this trial's own genuine, underlying sample size or connected statistical power

E. A p-value alone provides an entirely complete, sufficient statistical picture, with no genuine value from considering this same interval's own reported width

Answer: B. This genuinely wide confidence interval reflects genuine, limited precision in the trial's own effect estimate, meaning complete evaluation requires actively considering this interval's own width alongside the reported p-value, not either statistic in isolation.

This vignette directly tests this book's own foundational statistical inference content: correctly, precisely interpreting a genuinely current, specific 95 per cent confidence interval provides genuinely important, additional information beyond a given study's own, specific p-value alone.

This same interval directly reflects the genuine, precise range within which the true, actual effect genuinely, most plausibly lies, meaning correctly, completely evaluating a given study's own genuine result requires actively considering both this same interval's own genuine width, reflecting genuine precision, and its own genuine position relative to a given, clinically meaningful threshold.

This reflects this book's own repeated theme that correctly, critically appraising genuinely current evidence requires moving beyond a single, binary 'significant or not' interpretation alone, toward a genuinely richer, more complete statistical understanding — a genuinely wide interval directly signals genuine, remaining uncertainty regarding this same trial's own true, underlying effect size.

Why the other options are wrong

A. This wide interval carries direct, genuine relevance to correctly interpreting this result, as detailed in the correct answer.

C. A genuinely wide interval reflects genuinely different, less precise meaning compared with a genuinely narrow interval.

D. A direct, genuine relationship exists between interval width and sample size or statistical power.

E. Genuine, additional value exists from considering interval width, as detailed in the correct answer, not a p-value alone being sufficient.

Board Alert A genuinely wide 95 per cent confidence interval reflects genuine, limited precision in a trial's effect estimate, requiring active consideration alongside the reported p-value, not either statistic in isolation.

Question 41

A 26-week gestation infant with confirmed persistent pulmonary hypertension is being considered for ECMO at a referring, Level II facility. A specific, portable ECMO console is available. Which of the following best reflects the correct, honest risk-benefit consideration this circumstance requires?

A. Referring-centre cannulation carries no genuine, remaining risk of any kind, representing an unconditionally superior approach in every specific circumstance

B. Correctly, honestly weighing referring-centre cannulation against genuine, active transport followed by subsequent cannulation represents a genuinely important, honest risk-benefit consideration, since referring-centre cannulation directly avoids the genuine risk of significant, further deterioration during transport without extracorporeal support, while requiring this specific, technically demanding procedure to be performed away from a more familiar, specialised centre environment

C. Genuine, active transport followed by subsequent cannulation carries no genuine, meaningful risk of any kind

D. This specific risk-benefit consideration carries no genuine relevance to correctly, safely managing this specific circumstance

E. This procedure's own genuine degree of difficulty carries an identical, unchanged profile regardless of the specific location it is performed in

Answer: B. **Correctly, honestly weighing referring-centre cannulation against transport-then-cannulate represents a genuinely important risk-benefit consideration — avoiding**

unsupported transport deterioration, while requiring this demanding procedure away from a more familiar, specialised environment.

This vignette directly tests this book's own established transport and ECMO content: correctly, honestly weighing referring-centre cannulation against the alternative approach of genuine, active transport followed by subsequent cannulation at a specialised centre represents a genuinely important, honest risk-benefit consideration.

Referring-centre cannulation directly avoids the genuine risk of significant, further deterioration during transport without extracorporeal support, while this same approach nonetheless requires this specific, technically demanding procedure to be genuinely performed by a specialised team travelling to this infant, rather than within this infant's own, more familiar specialised centre environment.

This reflects this book's own repeated theme of honest, complete treatment of genuinely current clinical strategy, acknowledging that even a genuinely important, current technological advance carries its own, genuine trade-off requiring active, individual clinical judgment rather than a single, uniformly preferred approach.

Why the other options are wrong

A. A genuine, remaining risk-benefit consideration exists, as detailed in the correct answer, not an unconditionally superior approach.

C. A genuine, meaningful risk exists with this alternative approach, as detailed in the correct answer.

D. This specific consideration carries direct, essential relevance to safely managing this circumstance.

E. This procedure's own degree of difficulty genuinely differs based on location, as detailed in the correct answer.

Board Alert Referring-centre ECMO cannulation avoids unsupported transport deterioration but requires this technically demanding procedure to be performed away from a more familiar, specialised environment — a genuine, honest trade-off.

Mock Exam 2 — Section C: Application | Universal Task 4: Management, Treatment and Prevention

Question 42

A family whose infant has genuinely, actively been diagnosed with a significant, life-limiting condition asks the clinical team about the difference between palliative care and bereavement support, having heard both terms used somewhat interchangeably by different staff members. Which of the following best reflects the correct, complete, and clarifying response to this specific family question?

A. These two specific terms genuinely, correctly refer to an identical, single concept, with no meaningful, specific distinction between them

B. Palliative care, genuinely focused on maximising quality of life and genuine comfort throughout an infant's own, entire remaining life, however genuinely brief, is genuinely, specifically distinct from bereavement support, genuinely focused on directly supporting a family following this same infant's own actual death

C. Bereavement support genuinely, exclusively occurs before, rather than after, a given infant's own actual death

D. This specific distinction carries no genuine, meaningful relevance to correctly, appropriately supporting this family

E. This specific family question deserves no genuine, substantive, clarifying response of any kind

Answer: B. **Palliative care focuses on maximising quality of life throughout an infant's own remaining life, genuinely distinct from bereavement support, which directly supports a family following this infant's own actual death.**

This vignette directly tests this book's own foundational, and genuinely important, ethics distinction: palliative care, genuinely focused on maximising quality of life and genuine comfort throughout an infant's own, entire remaining life, however genuinely brief, is genuinely, specifically distinct from bereavement support, genuinely focused on directly, compassionately supporting a family following this same infant's own actual death.

This same, clarifying distinction directly ensures a given family receives correctly, appropriately tailored support at every genuine stage of this infant's own entire, connected clinical and, ultimately, bereavement journey, rather than confusion regarding which specific support this family is genuinely, currently receiving or should genuinely, actively seek.

This reflects this book's own repeated theme that this entire, genuinely sensitive field requires precise, careful attention to language and concept alike, not merely to clinical technique, since correctly, clearly explaining this specific distinction to a genuinely confused family represents a genuine act of compassionate, honest communication.

Why the other options are wrong

A. These reflect genuinely different, connected specific concepts, as detailed in the correct answer, not an identical concept.

C. This reverses the correct relationship; bereavement support genuinely occurs after, not before, this infant's own actual death.

D. This specific distinction carries direct, genuine relevance to appropriately supporting this family, as detailed in the correct answer.

E. This specific family question deserves a genuine, substantive, clarifying response, as detailed in the correct answer.

Board Alert Palliative care focuses on maximising quality of life throughout an infant's own remaining life. Bereavement support directly supports a family following this infant's own actual death — genuinely distinct, connected concepts.

Question 43

A genuinely current, specific quality improvement initiative reports a significant, measured improvement in a specific process measure — the proportion of eligible infants correctly screened for a specific condition — without reporting a corresponding change in the same infant population's own actual, longer-term clinical outcome. Which of the following best reflects the correct, complete interpretation of this specific finding?

A. A process measure and an outcome measure reflect an identical, single specific category, meaning this same improvement automatically, reliably confirms a corresponding improvement in this same outcome

B. This finding directly illustrates the genuine, important distinction between a process measure, reflecting whether a specific, intended action actually occurred, and an outcome measure, reflecting the actual, genuine clinical result this same action was ultimately intended to produce, meaning a genuinely improved process measure does not automatically, reliably guarantee a correspondingly improved outcome measure

C. This specific initiative's own reported finding carries no genuine, meaningful relevance to correctly, completely evaluating this same initiative's own actual effectiveness

D. An outcome measure carries no genuine, meaningful relationship to a process measure of any kind

E. This specific initiative should genuinely be considered an unconditional, complete success based on this single, reported process measure alone

Answer: B. **This finding illustrates the important distinction between a process measure (whether an action occurred) and an outcome measure (the actual clinical result) — a genuinely improved process measure does not automatically guarantee a correspondingly improved outcome measure.**

This vignette directly tests this book's own foundational quality improvement methodology content: a process measure, generally reflecting whether a specific, intended action or intervention actually, genuinely occurred, is genuinely, specifically distinct from an outcome measure, generally reflecting the actual, genuine clinical result this same action or intervention was ultimately intended to produce.

This means correctly, completely evaluating this specific quality improvement initiative requires actively tracking both of these genuinely different specific categories together, since a genuinely improved process measure does not automatically, reliably guarantee a correspondingly improved outcome measure, this specific gap in this vignette directly illustrating this same, important principle.

This reflects this book's own repeated theme that correctly, honestly evaluating a given quality improvement initiative requires structured, comprehensive measurement extending beyond a single, isolated metric alone, rather than assuming an improved process automatically translates into a correspondingly improved, genuine clinical outcome.

Why the other options are wrong

A. These reflect genuinely different, specific measurement categories, as detailed in the correct answer, not an identical category with automatic transfer.

C. This specific finding carries direct, genuine relevance to completely evaluating this initiative, as detailed in the correct answer.

D. A direct, genuine relationship exists between these two measures, though genuinely distinct, as detailed in the correct answer.

E. This finding does not automatically confirm unconditional success; further outcome evaluation is genuinely required.

Board Alert A process measure reflects whether an intended action occurred. An outcome measure reflects the actual clinical result. A genuinely improved process measure does not automatically guarantee a correspondingly improved outcome measure.

Question 44

A Level II neonatal intensive care unit is considering whether a genuinely current, specific research finding regarding a new intervention, developed and validated predominantly in extremely preterm infants at Level IV facilities, should genuinely be adopted for the more moderately preterm population this same unit predominantly serves. Which of the following best reflects the correct, critical consideration this specific circumstance requires?

A. This research finding should genuinely, automatically be adopted without any further, active consideration of any kind

B. This unit should actively consider this same study's own genuine, external validity, or generalisability, before adopting this specific intervention, since a given study's own finding, even when genuinely, internally valid, may genuinely not reliably generalise to a genuinely distinct population if this same population was genuinely, inadequately represented within this same, original study's own enrolled participants

C. This specific research finding carries no genuine relevance to correctly considering adoption at this specific unit

D. External validity carries no genuine, meaningful relevance to correctly considering this specific adoption decision

E. Every specific research finding genuinely, reliably generalises to every specific population regardless of this same population's own actual, original enrolment

Answer: B. **This unit should actively consider this study's own external validity before adopting this intervention, since a genuinely valid finding may not reliably generalise to this genuinely distinct, more moderately preterm population if**

inadequately represented in original enrolment.

This vignette directly tests this book's own established, closing biostatistics content: correctly, actively considering a given study's own genuine, external validity, or generalisability, particularly when applying a specific research finding to a genuinely distinct subpopulation, carries direct, genuine, connected importance.

This means a given study's own finding, even when genuinely, internally valid, may genuinely not, reliably generalise to this same, genuinely distinct subpopulation if this same subpopulation was genuinely, inadequately represented within this same, original study's own enrolled participants, this specific circumstance directly illustrating this same, important principle for the more moderately preterm population this unit predominantly serves.

This reflects this book's own repeated, closing theme that correctly, critically appraising genuinely current evidence requires active, final attention to whether a given study's own finding genuinely, reliably applies to the specific, individual population a given clinical team actually, genuinely cares for, rather than uncritical, automatic adoption regardless of this important, connected consideration.

Why the other options are wrong

A. Active, critical consideration is genuinely warranted, as detailed in the correct answer, not automatic adoption without evaluation.

C. This specific research finding carries direct, genuine relevance to this adoption decision, as detailed in the correct answer.

D. This specific consideration carries direct, essential relevance to this adoption decision, as detailed in the correct answer.

E. Genuine, meaningful variation in generalisability exists, not reliable generalisation regardless of enrolment.

Board Alert A given study's external validity requires active consideration before adopting an intervention for a genuinely distinct population — a genuinely valid finding may not reliably generalise if that population was inadequately represented in original enrolment.

Question 45

A Level III neonatal intensive care unit is developing a structured pre-transport checklist for infants requiring transfer to a Level IV facility. Which of the following combined elements would most directly reflect this book's own established, correct approach to safe, active neonatal transport?

A. A single, isolated checklist item alone, without any further, structured or combined component

B. Correctly, safely securing the airway and stable vascular access before movement actually begins, actively extending thermal management principles into this genuinely challenging, mobile environment, and applying permissive hypercapnia acid-base principles throughout, all coordinated through a structured, team-based communication process

C. This specific checklist requires no genuine, structured, coordinated, multidisciplinary development process of any kind

D. Thermal management principles carry no genuine relevance to this specific, mobile transport environment

E. This specific checklist can be correctly, safely developed without any genuine consideration of this book's own established acid-base content

Answer: B. **A correct, structured pre-transport checklist secures airway and vascular access before movement begins, extends thermal management principles into the mobile environment, applies permissive hypercapnia principles throughout, and is coordinated through structured, team-based communication.**

This vignette directly tests this book's own comprehensive transport content: correctly, safely securing the airway and stable vascular access before genuine, active transport actually begins is essential, since correction becomes considerably more difficult once movement has already begun — directly paralleling for both these specific, physiologic parameters.

This same transport directly requires actively, proactively extending this book's own extensively established thermal management principles into this specific, genuinely challenging mobile environment, and correctly, safely applying this book's own extensively established acid-base physiology principles, permissive hypercapnia specifically, to correctly, safely maintain appropriate ventilation throughout this same, mobile environment.

This reflects this book's own repeated theme that neonatal transport represents the genuinely comprehensive, structured extension of this book's own earlier, foundational content into a specific, mobile clinical environment, requiring a coordinated, structured pre-transport checklist directly extending this book's own repeated, coordinated care principle.

Why the other options are wrong

A. A single, isolated item does not reflect the genuinely comprehensive, combined approach this book establishes.

C. This checklist genuinely benefits from structured, coordinated, multidisciplinary development.

D. These principles carry direct, particular importance in this specific, mobile environment, as detailed in the correct answer.

E. This book's own established acid-base content carries direct, genuine relevance to this specific checklist.

Board Alert Safe neonatal transport requires securing airway and vascular access before movement begins, extending thermal management principles, applying permissive hypercapnia principles, and coordinated, structured team communication together.

Question 46

A family caring for an infant with a confirmed, significant, life-limiting genetic diagnosis expresses uncertainty about specific medical terminology used during a recent, difficult conversation with the clinical team. Which of the following best reflects the correct, compassionate response to this specific circumstance?

A. This family's own genuine confusion carries no genuine relevance to correctly, compassionately communicating with this family

B. Correctly, honestly acknowledging genuinely ambiguous terminology relating to this infant's own diagnosis or prognosis represents a genuinely important ethical consideration, meaning correctly, compassionately communicating with this family requires actively acknowledging genuine, remaining uncertainty in terminology itself, rather than presenting a genuinely ambiguous term as though it carried entirely clear, definitive meaning

C. This specific family's own confusion should genuinely be dismissed without any further, active, clarifying discussion

D. Medical terminology used in this specific context genuinely, always carries entirely clear, unambiguous meaning with no genuine, remaining uncertainty of any kind

E. This specific circumstance requires no further, active or honest communication of any kind with this family

Answer: B. Correctly, honestly acknowledging genuinely ambiguous terminology represents an important ethical consideration, requiring active acknowledgement of remaining uncertainty rather than presenting an ambiguous term as definitively clear.

This vignette directly tests this book's own established ethics content regarding specific, careful communication: correctly, honestly acknowledging genuinely ambiguous terminology relating to a given infant's own diagnosis or prognosis represents a specific, genuinely important ethical consideration directly extending this book's own repeated theme of honest, calibrated communication.

This means correctly, compassionately communicating with this family requires actively, deliberately acknowledging genuine, remaining uncertainty in terminology itself, rather than presenting a genuinely ambiguous term as though it carried entirely clear, definitive meaning, this same, honest acknowledgement directly addressing this family's own genuine, expressed confusion.

This reflects this book's own repeated theme that honest, complete communication requires attention not merely to what is genuinely known, but to what genuinely remains uncertain, even at the level of the specific language actually used, particularly when a family genuinely expresses this same, honest confusion.

Why the other options are wrong

A. This family's own confusion carries direct, essential relevance to correctly communicating with this family.

C. This confusion deserves active, honest, clarifying discussion, not dismissal, as detailed in the correct answer.

D. Genuine, remaining ambiguity can exist for certain specific terms, as detailed in the correct answer.

E. Active, honest communication is genuinely warranted in this specific circumstance.

Board Alert Correctly, honestly acknowledging genuinely ambiguous terminology relating to diagnosis or prognosis represents an important ethical consideration, requiring active acknowledgement of remaining uncertainty.

Question 47

A genuinely current guideline directly addresses ECMO training and continuing education for clinical staff. A newly hired neonatologist, having completed formal ECMO training 8 years prior at a different institution, asks whether this earlier training remains genuinely sufficient. Which of the following best reflects the correct, current understanding of this specific circumstance?

- **A.** This earlier, single training episode provides entirely sufficient, complete competency, with no genuine, further ongoing education required regardless of the time elapsed
- **B.** This genuinely current guideline directly reflects active, professional recognition that correctly, safely applying this technology requires ongoing, structured education rather than a single, initial training episode alone, meaning correctly, safely maintaining this specific clinical competency requires active, continuous professional development throughout an entire clinical career
- **C.** This specific question carries no genuine relevance to correctly, safely maintaining this clinical competency
- **D.** Ongoing, structured education carries no genuine, meaningful relevance to correctly, safely applying this specific technology
- **E.** This earlier training should genuinely be considered entirely invalid and require complete, full repetition from the very beginning

Answer: B. This genuinely current guideline reflects professional recognition that safe application requires ongoing, structured education rather than a single, initial episode — maintaining this competency requires active, continuous professional development throughout an entire clinical career.

This vignette directly tests this book's own established ECMO training content: a genuinely current, specific narrative guideline directly addresses ECMO training and continuing education, this genuinely current guideline directly reflecting active, professional recognition that correctly, safely applying this chapter's own central technology requires ongoing, structured education.

This means correctly, safely maintaining this specific clinical competency requires active, continuous professional development throughout an entire clinical career, rather than a single, initial training episode, however genuinely thorough at the time, being considered entirely, permanently sufficient regardless of the considerable time subsequently elapsed.

This reflects this book's own repeated theme that correctly, safely applying this chapter's own central technology requires not simply correct, initial technical knowledge, but active, ongoing professional maintenance of this same, genuinely demanding clinical skill set throughout an entire, ongoing career.

Why the other options are wrong

A. Active, ongoing education is genuinely required, as detailed in the correct answer, not a single, sufficient initial episode regardless of elapsed time.

C. This specific question carries direct, essential relevance to safely maintaining this competency.

D. This specific education carries direct, essential relevance to safely applying this technology, as detailed in the correct answer.

E. Complete repetition from the beginning is not specifically required; ongoing, structured continuing education is the correct approach.

Board Alert Genuinely current ECMO training guidelines reflect professional recognition that safe application requires ongoing, structured continuing education throughout an entire clinical career, not a single, initial training episode alone.

Question 48

A neonatal intensive care unit network spanning multiple states is developing a coordinated benchmarking initiative. Which of the following best reflects the correct, established rationale for this specific, broad, coordinated structure?

A. Isolated, single-facility improvement efforts provide an identical, equally effective approach compared with a coordinated, networked structure

B. Neonatal intensive care unit networks represent a specific, genuinely important platform for continuous quality improvement, since this same, broad, connected structure directly enables systematic benchmarking and structured, mutual, collaborative learning across multiple, genuinely distinct facilities together

C. This specific, coordinated structure carries no genuine, meaningful relevance to correctly, effectively improving neonatal outcomes

D. Benchmarking and collaborative learning carry no genuine, meaningful relationship to this specific, networked structure

E. A genuinely broad, coordinated structure carries no genuine advantage over a single, isolated facility acting independently

Answer: B. **Neonatal intensive care unit networks represent a genuinely important platform for continuous quality improvement, enabling systematic benchmarking and structured, collaborative learning across multiple, genuinely distinct facilities together.**

This vignette directly tests this book's own established care systems content: neonatal intensive care unit networks, spanning genuinely broad regions, states, or entire countries together, represent a specific, genuinely important platform for continuous quality improvement.

This same, broad, connected structure directly enables systematic benchmarking, structured identification and implementation of best available evidence, and structured, mutual, collaborative learning across multiple, genuinely distinct facilities together, this same, coordinated approach directly reflecting this book's own repeated theme regarding coordinated, connected expertise.

This reflects this book's own repeated, closing theme that safe, effective neonatal care depends not simply on individual clinical decision-making or even single-facility quality improvement alone, but on the broader, coordinated, networked systems within which this same care is actually delivered.

Why the other options are wrong

A. A coordinated, networked structure provides genuinely superior, not identical, outcome improvement compared with isolated efforts.

C. This specific structure carries direct, genuine relevance to improving outcomes, as detailed in the correct answer.

D. A direct, essential relationship exists between these activities and this specific structure, as detailed in the correct answer.

E. This broad, coordinated structure provides genuine, established advantage over a single, isolated facility, as detailed in the correct answer.

Board Alert Neonatal intensive care unit networks represent a genuinely important platform for continuous quality improvement, enabling systematic benchmarking and structured, collaborative learning across multiple facilities.

Question 49

A genuinely current, specific meta-analysis pools data from twelve individual randomised controlled trials examining a common perinatal intervention. Which of the following best reflects a genuinely important, connected limitation this specific study design requires active, critical consideration of?

A. This specific study design carries no genuine, connected limitation of any kind, providing entirely, definitively conclusive evidence

B. Publication bias, reflecting the genuine tendency for studies demonstrating a genuinely positive, significant result to be genuinely, more likely published than studies demonstrating a genuinely negative or null result, means this same meta-analysis genuinely, potentially risks overestimating the true, actual effect if this same, underlying bias genuinely exists within this same field's own published literature

C. This specific limitation carries no genuine, meaningful relevance to correctly interpreting this specific meta-analysis

D. Studies demonstrating a genuinely negative or null result are genuinely, more likely to be published than studies demonstrating a genuinely positive, significant result

E. A meta-analysis carries no genuine, potential risk of overestimating a given, true effect of any kind

Answer: B. **Publication bias, reflecting the genuine tendency for positive, significant studies to be more likely published, means this meta-analysis genuinely risks overestimating the true effect if this bias genuinely exists within this field's published literature.**

This vignette directly tests this book's own established biostatistics content regarding systematic review and meta-analysis: publication bias represents a genuinely important, specific limitation directly relevant to this specific, combined study design, reflecting the genuine tendency for studies demonstrating a genuinely positive, significant result to be genuinely, more likely published.

This means this same meta-analysis genuinely, potentially risks overestimating a given, true effect if this same, underlying publication bias genuinely, actually exists within this same, specific field's own published literature, reinforcing this book's own repeated theme that even a genuinely stronger, more powerful study design carries its own, genuine, specific limitation.

This reflects this book's own repeated theme that correctly, critically appraising even this book's own, most powerful specific study design requires active, ongoing attention to this same design's own genuine, specific limitation, rather than treating a meta-analysis as automatically, definitively conclusive regardless of this important, connected consideration.

Why the other options are wrong

A. A genuine, connected limitation exists, as detailed in the correct answer, not entirely, definitively conclusive evidence.

C. This specific limitation carries direct, essential relevance to correctly interpreting this meta-analysis.

D. This reverses the correct relationship; positive, significant studies, not negative or null studies, are genuinely more likely published.

E. A genuine, potential risk of overestimation exists, as detailed in the correct answer.

Board Alert Publication bias — the genuine tendency for positive, significant studies to be more likely published — means a meta-analysis genuinely risks overestimating a true effect if this bias exists within the field's published literature.

Mock Exam 2 — Section C: Application | Universal Task 4: Management, Treatment and Prevention

Question 50

A term infant with confirmed, severe meconium aspiration syndrome and secondary persistent pulmonary hypertension, genuinely failing maximal conventional therapy, is being evaluated for ECMO at a referring centre. Which of the following configurations is generally favoured, and what genuinely current technological consideration is also directly relevant to this specific circumstance?

A. Venoarterial configuration is generally favoured, and genuinely current technology carries no genuine relevance to this specific circumstance

B. Venovenous configuration is generally favoured, given this infant's own predominantly respiratory pathology, and genuinely current technology may enable safe cannulation at this referring centre before transport, requiring the specialised, coordinated mobile ECMO team this circumstance directly demands

C. Neither configuration carries any genuine, meaningful distinction relevant to this specific clinical decision

D. This infant's own specific respiratory pathology carries no genuine relevance to correctly selecting an appropriate configuration

E. Genuinely current technology carries no genuine relevance to correctly planning this infant's own specific transport and ECMO approach

> **Answer: B. Venovenous configuration is generally favoured given this infant's predominantly respiratory pathology, and genuinely current technology may enable safe cannulation at this referring centre before transport, requiring the specialised, coordinated mobile ECMO team this circumstance demands.**
>
> This vignette directly tests this book's own established ECMO content together: confirmed, severe meconium aspiration syndrome with secondary persistent pulmonary hypertension, genuinely failing maximal therapy, represents a genuinely important, connected respiratory indication, generally favouring venovenous configuration given this infant's own predominantly respiratory pathology.
>
> This same circumstance directly connects to this book's own genuinely current technological content: genuinely current technology may enable safe cannulation at this referring facility before transport begins, requiring the specialised, coordinated mobile ECMO team this circumstance directly demands, rather than reflexively assuming transport must always precede this specific technology.
>
> This reflects this book's own repeated theme that correct, complete management of this genuinely complex circumstance requires synthesising foundational configuration selection together with genuinely current, evolving technological and logistical considerations, rather than treating either consideration in complete isolation from the other.

Why the other options are wrong

A. Venovenous, not venoarterial, configuration is generally favoured given this predominantly respiratory pathology; technology is directly relevant.

C. A genuinely important, meaningful distinction exists between these two configurations, as detailed in the correct answer.

D. This infant's own respiratory pathology carries direct, essential relevance to selecting the appropriate configuration.

E. This genuinely current technology carries direct, genuine relevance to planning this specific approach, as detailed in the correct answer.

Board Alert Meconium aspiration syndrome with secondary pulmonary hypertension generally favours venovenous configuration. Genuinely current, portable technology may enable safe, on-site cannulation before transport.

Question 51

A 28-week gestation infant develops significant, progressive abdominal distension with feeding intolerance. A specific 2025 externally-validated nomogram incorporating clinical and laboratory parameters is applied to estimate this infant's own risk of postoperative intestinal failure or death should surgical intervention become necessary. Which of the following best reflects the correct, honest understanding of this specific tool's own genuine, clinical role?

A. This specific nomogram carries no genuine, established basis in current, published literature of any kind

B. This genuinely current, externally-validated nomogram provides genuinely important, quantified, individualised risk information directly supporting more informed, structured family counselling and clinical decision-making, though this same tool's own genuine, current predictive accuracy should be actively, honestly considered alongside a given infant's own broader, individual clinical circumstance

C. This specific tool provides entirely complete, sufficient information on its own, with no genuine need for any further, active clinical judgment

D. This specific tool carries no genuine relevance to correctly counselling this infant's own family

E. This specific tool has already achieved entirely, universally perfect predictive accuracy across every specific circumstance

Answer: B. This genuinely current, externally-validated nomogram provides important, quantified, individualised risk information supporting informed counselling and decision-making, though its predictive accuracy should be honestly considered alongside this infant's broader, individual circumstance.

This vignette directly tests this book's own established surgical content: a genuinely current, December 2025, externally-validated nomogram for postoperative intestinal failure or death directly represents a genuinely important, quantified tool supporting structured, informed family counselling and clinical decision-making in necrotising enterocolitis.

This same, genuinely current tool provides genuinely important, individualised, quantified risk information, directly enhancing correctly, compassionately informed shared decision-making conversations with this infant's own family, reflecting this book's own repeated theme regarding the genuine, practical value of structured, evidence-based tools.

This reflects this book's own repeated theme of honest evidence treatment: even a genuinely current, externally-validated tool should be actively, honestly considered alongside a given infant's own broader, individual clinical circumstance, rather than treated as an entirely complete, infallible substitute for ongoing, integrated clinical judgment.

Why the other options are wrong

A. This specific tool has direct, genuine basis in current, published literature, as detailed in the correct answer.

C. Active, ongoing clinical judgment remains genuinely necessary alongside this specific tool, as detailed in the correct answer.

D. This specific tool carries direct, genuine relevance to counselling this family, as detailed in the correct answer.

E. Genuine, honest consideration of this tool's own accuracy remains warranted, not assumption of universally perfect accuracy.

Board Alert A genuinely current, externally-validated nomogram for postoperative intestinal failure or death in necrotising enterocolitis supports informed counselling, though should be considered alongside a given infant's own broader clinical circumstance.

Question 52

A 27-week gestation infant is 5 weeks old and has demonstrated evolving, significant, cystic changes on cranial ultrasound in the periventricular white matter. Which of the following best reflects the correct, comprehensive approach to counselling this infant's family regarding this specific finding?

A. This family should genuinely be provided with no specific, substantive information regarding this finding's own significance

B. This family deserves honest, complete counselling that this finding reflects significant white matter injury carrying genuine, established relevance to this infant's own longer-term neurodevelopmental outcome, including elevated cerebral palsy risk, together with active, genuine commitment to structured, longer-term follow-up monitoring this same, connected trajectory

C. This finding carries no genuine, established relevance to this infant's own longer-term outcome of any kind

D. This family should genuinely be told this finding will definitely, completely resolve without any genuine, lasting consequence

E. This specific finding requires no further, structured or connected follow-up of any kind

Answer: B. **This family deserves honest counselling that this finding reflects significant white matter injury with genuine, established relevance to longer-term outcome, including elevated cerebral palsy risk, together with genuine commitment to structured, longer-term follow-up.**

This vignette directly tests this book's own established neurology and honest communication content together: cystic periventricular leukomalacia reflects genuine, significant white matter injury, carrying established, connected relevance to this infant's own longer-term neurodevelopmental trajectory, including a genuinely elevated risk of cerebral palsy.

This same, honest finding directly supports the same structured, longer-term neurodevelopmental follow-up programme this book has established repeatedly throughout its own content as essential for this high-risk population, extending clinical attention well beyond the acute, immediate neonatal period alone.

This reflects this book's own repeated theme that honest, complete communication with a family requires actively, honestly sharing genuinely significant, connected findings, together with a clear, concrete, and genuinely reassuring plan for ongoing, structured, and connected clinical attention, rather than either withholding significant information or offering false, complete reassurance.

Why the other options are wrong

A. This family deserves genuine, substantive, honest information regarding this finding, as detailed in the correct answer.

C. A direct, well-established relationship exists between this finding and this infant's own longer-term outcome.

D. This finding carries genuine, established, potentially lasting consequence; false, complete reassurance is not appropriate.

E. Structured, longer-term follow-up is genuinely warranted for this specific finding, as detailed in the correct answer.

Board Alert Cystic periventricular leukomalacia requires honest counselling regarding genuine, established longer-term neurodevelopmental relevance, including elevated cerebral palsy risk, together with structured, longer-term follow-up.

Question 53

A term infant is noted at birth to have a large, midline abdominal wall defect covered by a membranous sac, with visible liver and bowel within this same sac. Which of the following best reflects the correct, immediate diagnostic and connected consideration this specific presentation requires?

A. This presentation is most consistent with gastroschisis, requiring no further, connected evaluation of any kind

B. This presentation is most consistent with omphalocele, given the presence of a covering membrane, and this finding should prompt active evaluation for connected chromosomal and cardiac anomalies, given this specific condition's own genuinely elevated, established association with these further, connected findings

C. The presence of a covering membrane carries no genuine, diagnostic significance in distinguishing between these two specific conditions

D. This presentation carries no genuine, established relationship to any further, connected structural or chromosomal anomaly

E. This specific condition requires no further, active evaluation or connected management of any kind

Answer: B. **This presentation is most consistent with omphalocele, given the presence of a covering membrane, which should prompt active evaluation for connected chromosomal and cardiac anomalies, given this condition's genuinely elevated, established association.**

This vignette directly tests this book's own established surgical distinction: omphalocele, genuinely distinct from gastroschisis, is specifically characterised by the presence of a covering membrane, this same, defining feature directly present in this infant's own specific description.

This specific condition carries a genuinely elevated, established association with connected chromosomal and cardiac anomalies, genuinely distinct from gastroschisis's own, more genuinely elevated association with bowel injury, atresia, and fluid loss instead — this book's own repeated theme regarding correctly, precisely distinguishing between two genuinely similar-appearing conditions.

This means correctly, completely evaluating this infant requires active, structured evaluation for these further, connected anomalies, rather than assuming this infant's own presentation, however structurally significant, represents an entirely isolated, unconnected finding.

Why the other options are wrong

A. The presence of a covering membrane is more consistent with omphalocele, not gastroschisis, which lacks this membrane.

C. This specific feature carries direct, established diagnostic significance in distinguishing these two conditions.

D. A direct, established, elevated association exists with these further, connected anomalies, as detailed in the correct answer.

E. Active, structured evaluation for connected anomalies is genuinely warranted for this specific condition.

> **Board Alert** Omphalocele, characterised by a covering membrane, carries a genuinely elevated, established association with connected chromosomal and cardiac anomalies, distinct from gastroschisis's own connected risk profile.

Question 54

A 25-week gestation infant is 3 weeks old and is undergoing genuinely current, routine neuromonitoring while receiving ECMO support. A genuinely current, externally-validated machine learning model is being used alongside standard monitoring to help predict this infant's own risk of significant brain injury. Which of the following best reflects the correct, honest understanding of this specific tool's own genuine role?

A. This specific model carries no genuine, established basis in genuinely current, published research of any kind

B. This genuinely current, externally-validated machine learning model represents a genuinely important, complementary tool directly supporting this book's own established routine neuromonitoring guideline content, meaning correctly, completely understanding this infant's own connected neurological risk requires actively considering multiple, genuinely distinct, current research approaches together, rather than any single, isolated tool alone

C. This specific model provides an entirely complete, sufficient neurological assessment on its own, with no genuine need for any further, structured monitoring

D. This specific tool carries no genuine relevance to correctly, safely managing an infant supported on this specific technology

E. Machine learning models carry no genuine, established role in genuinely current neonatal ECMO research of any kind

> **Answer: B. This genuinely current, externally-validated machine learning model represents an important, complementary tool supporting this book's own routine neuromonitoring guideline content, requiring consideration of multiple, distinct approaches together, not any single, isolated tool alone.**
>
> This vignette directly tests this book's own genuinely current ECMO neuromonitoring content: genuinely current guidelines address routine neuromonitoring, complemented by a genuinely current, externally validated

machine learning model directly, specifically identified as a further, connected research approach to this same, important clinical concern.

This means correctly, completely understanding this infant's own connected neurological risk requires actively, deliberately considering multiple, genuinely distinct, current research approaches together, reinforcing this chapter's repeated theme that genuinely current, active research continues to address this technology's own connected neurological risk from multiple, genuinely complementary, methodological directions.

This reflects this book's own repeated theme that a genuinely current, sophisticated tool represents a genuinely important, complementary addition to, rather than a complete, sufficient replacement for, this book's own established, structured neuromonitoring guideline content.

Why the other options are wrong

A. This specific model has direct, genuine basis in current, published research, as detailed in the correct answer.

C. This model complements, rather than entirely replaces, structured monitoring, as detailed in the correct answer.

D. This specific tool carries direct, genuine relevance to safely managing this infant, as detailed in the correct answer.

E. A genuine, established role exists for this specific technology in current research, as detailed in the correct answer.

Board Alert Genuinely current guidelines address routine ECMO neuromonitoring, complemented by an externally validated machine learning model — multiple, distinct research approaches together, not any single, isolated tool alone.

Mock Exam 2 — Section B: Organ Systems | Universal Task 3: Diagnosis, Testing and Monitoring

Question 55

A term infant born to a mother with confirmed, active Group B Streptococcus colonization who received inadequate intrapartum antibiotic prophylaxis develops significant respiratory distress and temperature instability within the first 6 hours of life. Which of the following represents the most appropriate, immediate approach?

A. No further, active evaluation is genuinely warranted, given this infant's own currently stable, initial appearance

B. This infant's presentation, combined with inadequate maternal intrapartum prophylaxis for confirmed Group B Streptococcus colonization, should prompt active, prompt evaluation for early-onset sepsis, including blood culture and empiric antibiotic therapy, given this specific, elevated risk profile

C. This infant's presentation carries no genuine, connected relationship to this specific maternal colonization history

D. This infant should genuinely receive no further, active monitoring following this initial evaluation, regardless of this infant's own subsequent clinical course

E. Maternal intrapartum antibiotic prophylaxis adequacy carries no genuine relevance to correctly evaluating this specific infant

Answer: B. This presentation, combined with inadequate maternal intrapartum prophylaxis for confirmed GBS colonization, should prompt active, prompt evaluation for early-onset sepsis, including blood culture and empiric antibiotic therapy, given this elevated risk profile.

This vignette directly tests this book's own established infectious disease content regarding early-onset Group B Streptococcus sepsis risk: this infant's own significant, new respiratory distress and temperature instability, combined with confirmed maternal colonization and inadequate intrapartum antibiotic prophylaxis, together represent a genuinely elevated, connected risk profile for early-onset sepsis.

Correct, immediate management directly requires active, prompt evaluation, including blood culture, together with empiric antibiotic therapy pending these same results, this specific approach directly reflecting this book's own repeated theme that correctly, actively recognising a specific, elevated risk profile directly changes the appropriate, immediate management approach.

This reflects this book's own repeated theme that correctly, safely evaluating a genuinely at-risk infant requires actively integrating maternal risk factors together with this infant's own specific, presenting clinical findings, rather than either specific consideration evaluated in complete isolation from the other.

Why the other options are wrong

A. This infant's own elevated, connected risk profile warrants active evaluation, not an absence of further consideration.

C. This presentation carries direct, connected relevance to this maternal colonization history, as detailed in the correct answer.

D. Active, ongoing monitoring remains genuinely warranted following this initial evaluation.

E. This specific adequacy carries direct, essential relevance to correctly evaluating this infant.

Board Alert Respiratory distress and temperature instability, combined with confirmed maternal GBS colonization and inadequate intrapartum prophylaxis, should prompt active evaluation for early-onset sepsis with blood culture and empiric antibiotics.

Question 56

A 24-week gestation infant is 1 week old and is being managed with a structured pain and sedation scoring tool. The clinical team is also actively applying developmental pharmacokinetic principles to guide analgesic dosing. Which of the following best reflects the correct, connected rationale for combining these two specific approaches?

A. These two specific approaches carry an identical, single function, with no meaningful, specific distinction between them

B. Correctly, safely managing sedation and analgesia in this specific population requires actively combining a structured, objective assessment tool with active, individualised application of this population's own genuinely distinctive developmental pharmacokinetics, since neither approach alone provides an entirely complete, sufficient basis for safe, correct clinical management

C. This infant's own specific gestational age carries no genuine relevance to correctly combining these two specific approaches

D. A structured scoring tool alone provides an entirely complete, sufficient basis for correct, safe clinical management

E. Developmental pharmacokinetic principles carry no genuine relevance to correctly, safely managing sedation and analgesia

Answer: B. **Correctly managing sedation and analgesia requires**

actively combining a structured, objective assessment tool with individualised application of developmental pharmacokinetics, since neither approach alone provides a complete, sufficient basis for safe management.

This vignette directly tests this book's own established pharmacology content: correctly, actively using a specific, validated pain and sedation scoring tool provides a genuinely important, structured, and considerably more objective approach to guiding sedation and analgesia decisions than clinical impression alone.

This same, structured approach directly requires active application of this book's own extensively established developmental pharmacokinetic principles — this population's own genuinely distinctive drug handling, reduced hepatic blood flow, and receptor and enzyme ontogeny together — since correctly, safely dosing a given medication genuinely requires both accurate assessment and individually appropriate dosing together.

This reflects this book's own repeated theme that correctly, safely applying sedation and analgesia in this genuinely vulnerable population requires both structured, objective clinical assessment and active, individualised, developmentally aware pharmacological judgment together, neither approach alone providing an entirely complete, sufficient basis for safe management.

Why the other options are wrong

A. These reflect genuinely different, complementary specific functions, as detailed in the correct answer, not an identical function.

C. This infant's own gestational age carries direct, essential relevance to combining these two approaches.

D. A scoring tool alone provides an incomplete basis; individualised pharmacokinetic application is also genuinely required.

E. These principles carry direct, essential relevance to safely managing sedation and analgesia, as detailed in the correct answer.

Board Alert Correctly managing procedural sedation and analgesia requires combining a structured, objective assessment tool with individualised developmental pharmacokinetic principles — neither approach alone is sufficient.

Question 57

A term infant develops significant, progressive abdominal distension and bilious vomiting beginning on day 3 of life, with a prior history of normal meconium passage in the first 24 hours. Contrast enema demonstrates a specific, characteristic transition zone in the distal colon. Which of the following best reflects the most likely, underlying diagnosis?

A. This presentation carries no genuine, connected relationship to any specific, recognised surgical diagnosis

B. This presentation is most consistent with Hirschsprung disease, this specific transition zone directly reflecting the genuine, connected boundary between the aganglionic segment and the more proximal, normally innervated bowel

C. This presentation is most consistent with intestinal malrotation with volvulus, which does not characteristically demonstrate this specific radiographic finding

D. A contrast enema carries no genuine, diagnostic utility in evaluating this specific presentation

E. This infant's own prior, normal meconium passage definitively excludes any further, active diagnostic consideration

Answer: B. **This presentation is most consistent with Hirschsprung disease, this specific transition zone directly reflecting the genuine, connected boundary between the aganglionic segment and the more proximal, normally innervated bowel.**

This vignette directly tests this book's own established surgical content regarding Hirschsprung disease's own characteristic radiographic finding: a specific, characteristic transition zone on contrast enema directly reflects the genuine, connected anatomic boundary between the distal, aganglionic segment and the more proximal, normally innervated, and consequently dilated, bowel.

This infant's own prior, normal meconium passage does not entirely, definitively exclude this diagnosis, since Hirschsprung disease can genuinely present with a more delayed, variable onset of symptoms, this specific presentation directly illustrating this book's own repeated theme regarding genuine variability in presentation timing for a given, connected condition.

This reflects this book's own repeated theme that correctly, precisely recognising a specific, characteristic radiographic finding directly supports confirmatory diagnosis, typically requiring rectal biopsy demonstrating genuine, confirmed absence of ganglion cells, before proceeding to definitive, surgical management.

Why the other options are wrong

A. A direct, well-established, connected relationship exists between this presentation and this specific, recognised diagnosis.

C. This specific radiographic finding is characteristic of Hirschsprung disease, not intestinal malrotation with volvulus.

D. This imaging modality carries direct, established diagnostic utility in evaluating this specific presentation.

E. This prior finding does not entirely, definitively exclude this diagnosis, as detailed in the correct answer.

Board Alert A characteristic transition zone on contrast enema directly reflects Hirschsprung disease's connected boundary between the aganglionic segment and the more proximal, normally innervated, dilated bowel.

Question 58

A 26-week gestation infant is being evaluated for possible extremely preterm ECMO candidacy given confirmed, severe respiratory failure. The clinical team calculates this infant's own oxygenation index as part of this evaluation. Which of the following best reflects the correct, connected understanding of this specific calculation's own genuine clinical role?

A. The oxygenation index carries no genuine, specific relationship to correctly determining ECMO candidacy of any kind

B. The oxygenation index, directly incorporating mean airway pressure, fraction of inspired oxygen, and arterial oxygen tension together, provides a specific, quantified measure of the genuine severity of this infant's own respiratory failure, directly, quantitatively informing correctly, appropriately determining whether this infant genuinely meets established candidacy criteria

C. Mean airway pressure and fraction of inspired oxygen carry no genuine, mechanistic relationship to this specific calculated parameter

D. Unstructured, purely subjective clinical impression represents the genuinely preferred, superior approach compared with this specific, calculated parameter

E. This specific parameter carries no genuine, quantitative relevance to correctly determining candidacy of any kind

Answer: B. The oxygenation index, incorporating mean airway pressure, fraction of inspired oxygen, and arterial oxygen tension together, provides a specific, quantified measure of respiratory failure severity, directly informing appropriate ECMO candidacy determination.

This vignette directly tests this book's own established ECMO fundamentals content: the oxygenation index, a specific, calculated parameter directly incorporating mean airway pressure, fraction of inspired oxygen, and arterial oxygen tension together, provides a specific, quantified measure of the genuine severity of a given infant's own respiratory failure.

This means this specific, calculated parameter directly, quantitatively informs correctly, appropriately determining whether a given infant genuinely meets established candidacy criteria for this chapter's own central technology, rather than relying on unstructured, purely subjective clinical impression alone.

This reflects this book's own repeated theme that correctly, safely applying this chapter's own central technology requires structured, quantitative assessment directly informing this genuinely important clinical decision, this same structured approach directly relevant to this infant's own genuinely challenging, extremely preterm candidacy evaluation.

Why the other options are wrong

A. A direct, well-established relationship exists, as detailed in the correct answer, not an absence of relationship.

C. These specific factors have a direct, defining relationship to this calculation, as detailed in the correct answer.

D. This specific, structured parameter provides genuinely superior, not inferior, guidance compared with subjective impression alone.

E. This specific parameter carries direct, quantitative relevance to determining candidacy, as detailed in the correct answer.

Board Alert The oxygenation index, incorporating mean airway pressure, fraction of inspired oxygen, and arterial oxygen tension together, provides a quantified measure of respiratory failure severity directly informing ECMO candidacy.

Question 59

A genuinely current, specific randomised controlled trial enrolling extremely preterm infants reports an intention-to-treat analysis alongside a separate, per-protocol analysis, with the two analyses yielding somewhat different, connected results. Which of the following best reflects the correct, critical appraisal this specific divergence requires?

- **A.** These two, genuinely distinct analytical approaches always, reliably produce an identical, single result, making this described divergence inaccurate
- **B.** This divergence directly reflects the genuine, established distinction between an intention-to-treat analysis, including every specific participant according to their own original, randomised assignment regardless of adherence, and a per-protocol analysis, including only participants genuinely completing this study as intended, with the intention-to-treat analysis generally preserving this trial's own randomisation-derived balance more genuinely
- **C.** This specific divergence carries no genuine, meaningful relevance to correctly, critically appraising this specific trial
- **D.** A per-protocol analysis generally preserves this trial's own randomisation-derived balance more genuinely than an intention-to-treat analysis
- **E.** This specific divergence has no established basis in genuinely current, recognised biostatistics literature of any kind

Answer: B. This divergence reflects the genuine, established distinction between an intention-to-treat analysis, including every participant by original assignment, and a per-protocol analysis, including only those completing as intended — with intention-to-treat generally preserving randomisation-derived balance more genuinely.

This vignette directly tests this book's own established biostatistics content: an intention-to-treat analysis, in which every specific participant is genuinely, actively analysed according to their own original, randomised assignment regardless of genuine, actual adherence, is genuinely, specifically distinct from a per-protocol analysis, in which only participants genuinely, actually completing this same, specific study according to this same, original protocol are genuinely, actively included.

This means an intention-to-treat analysis generally, more genuinely preserves this same, original trial's own randomisation-derived, genuine balance, this same, genuine distinction directly explaining why these two, genuinely different specific analytical approaches can genuinely produce somewhat different, connected results.

This reflects this book's own repeated theme that correctly, critically interpreting a given randomised trial requires actively considering which of these two, genuinely distinct analytical approaches this same trial actually, genuinely applied and reported, directly connecting to this book's own broader, honest evidence-treatment theme regarding missing outcome data and genuine adherence.

Why the other options are wrong

A. These two approaches can genuinely, meaningfully differ, as detailed in the correct answer, not always producing an identical result.

C. This specific divergence carries direct, essential relevance to critically appraising this trial, as detailed in the correct answer.

D. This reverses the correct relationship; an intention-to-treat, not per-protocol, analysis more genuinely preserves this balance.

E. This specific divergence has direct, genuine basis in genuinely current, recognised biostatistics literature.

Board Alert An intention-to-treat analysis includes every participant by original assignment regardless of adherence, generally preserving a trial's randomisation-derived balance more genuinely than a per-protocol analysis, which includes only those completing as intended.

Question 60

This is the final question of Mock Exam 2. A 25-week gestation, small-for-gestational-age infant is 6 weeks old and remains critically ill with evolving bronchopulmonary dysplasia, a recently confirmed grade III intraventricular haemorrhage, and a structured iron deficiency screening evaluation currently underway. The family is meeting with a coordinated, multidisciplinary team to discuss this infant's own overall trajectory and ongoing care. Which of the following best reflects the complete, correct, and coordinated approach to this entire, connected circumstance?

A. Each specific finding should genuinely be addressed by an entirely separate, unconnected clinical team, without any genuine, coordinated, shared discussion with this family

B. Recognise that this infant's evolving bronchopulmonary dysplasia reflects this book's own established, bidirectional and multifactorial risk framework, requiring careful, ongoing ventilator and acid-base management; recognise that this infant's confirmed grade III intraventricular haemorrhage carries genuine, established relevance to longer-term neurodevelopmental outcome, requiring the same structured, longer-term follow-up this book establishes as essential; recognise that this infant's iron deficiency screening carries genuine, connected relevance to neuroprotection; and recognise that this family deserves the same honest, shared decision-making conversation, honestly incorporating all of this connected, genuine uncertainty, that this entire book has modelled throughout its complete, five-volume span

C. This infant's own multiple, connected findings carry no genuine relationship to one another, requiring entirely separate, unconnected evaluation

D. This family's own genuine values and preferences carry no genuine relevance to this specific, coordinated conversation

E. This genuinely complex, multi-system circumstance can be correctly, completely managed without any genuine, coordinated, multidisciplinary discussion of any kind

Answer: B. **Every principle across this entire exam converges here: the bidirectional, multifactorial BPD risk framework, the connected neurodevelopmental relevance of significant IVH, the connected neuroprotective relevance of iron screening, and the honest, shared decision-making conversation this family deserves throughout.**

This truly final question of Mock Exam 2 is deliberately constructed to require synthesis across essentially every domain this exam has addressed — foundations, organ systems, and application together — mirroring the equivalent final integrative questions constructed throughout this entire book.

This infant's evolving bronchopulmonary dysplasia directly reflects this book's own established, bidirectional and multifactorial risk framework; this infant's confirmed grade III intraventricular haemorrhage carries genuine, established relevance to longer-term neurodevelopmental outcome, requiring the same structured, longer-term follow-up established throughout this book; and this infant's ongoing iron deficiency screening carries genuine, connected relevance to neuroprotection, directly connecting a haematological quality improvement target to this infant's own broader, connected developmental trajectory.

This family deserves the same honest, shared decision-making conversation, honestly incorporating all of this connected, genuine uncertainty, that this entire book has modelled throughout its complete, five-volume span, closing this exam on precisely the standard of connected, compassionate synthesis this entire project has been built toward.

Why the other options are wrong

A. A genuine, coordinated, shared discussion, not entirely separate, unconnected teams, represents the correct approach.

C. These findings are directly, mechanistically connected to one another, as detailed in the correct answer.

D. This family's own genuine values carry direct, essential relevance to this conversation, as detailed in the correct answer.

E. This genuinely complex circumstance requires coordinated, multidisciplinary discussion, not an absence of this coordination.

Board Alert This is the truly final question of Mock Exam 2, deliberately constructed to require synthesis of bronchopulmonary dysplasia risk, significant IVH follow-up, connected neuroprotective screening, and honest, shared family communication together.

Score Tracker: Mock Examination 2

Record your score by section below, and directly compare against your Mock Examination 1 result for each section.

Reflection Prompts

Did your weakest section change between the two exams, or stay the same? A persistent weak section is the clearest, most reliable signal of where focused revision will have the greatest, genuine impact.

For any question testing a critical appraisal skill — interpreting a confidence interval, distinguishing intention-to-treat from per-protocol analysis, weighing external validity — return to Volume 4's biostatistics chapter directly, since this reasoning pattern recurs throughout the actual certifying examination.

One further mock examination remains after this one, followed by the reference ranges appendix that closes out this entire book.

Mock Examination 3

The Final Practice Examination in This Series

60 Questions — Foundations, Organ Systems, and Application Together

A Third, Genuinely Independent Set of Vignettes

As with Mock Examinations 1 and 2, every question here is newly written and independent of the other two exams. This third exam leans further into differential diagnosis and connected, multi-step reasoning — several questions present an evolving clinical picture (a finding that changes over hours or days) rather than a single, static snapshot, and several deliberately connect two or three findings across different organ systems in a single infant, mirroring how real, complex neonatal presentations actually unfold.

The final question of this exam is also the final question of this entire, five-volume question bank. It draws together nearly every major theme this book has built across its complete span — physiological foundation, organ-system pathophysiology, surgical and technological application, honest evidence appraisal, and compassionate, shared communication — into a single, connected clinical circumstance, exactly as the real certifying examination, and real clinical practice, ultimately demand.

How to Use This Exam

If you have completed Mock Examinations 1 and 2, this is the natural final step before turning to the reference ranges appendix that closes out this book.

Work through all 60 questions in a single, timed sitting if possible, targeting roughly 90 seconds per question.

After finishing, look back across all three mock examinations together. A section that was weak in all three is the single clearest signal in this entire book of where your remaining preparation time will do the most good.

A Note on Figures

Every figure in this book is original artwork, drawn specifically for it. No stock images, no licensed photographs and no third-party illustrations are used anywhere in the text.

Questions

Section A: Foundations (Questions 1-9) — Section B: Organ Systems (Questions 10–58) — Section C: Application (Questions 28, 34–35, 40, 48–49, 51, 55, 57, 59–60)

Mock Exam 3 — Section A: Foundations | Universal Task 4: Management, Treatment and Prevention

Question 1

A 23-week gestation fetus is expected to deliver within the next 48 hours. The family has completed antenatal counselling and elected active resuscitation. At delivery, the infant is limp, apnoeic, and bradycardic. The cord has not yet been clamped, and the necessary equipment for deferred clamping is genuinely available. Which of the following represents the correct, immediate sequence of steps?

A. Immediately clamp and cut the cord, then transfer to the warmer before any further assessment

B. Begin initial steps and positive pressure ventilation as needed while genuinely deferring cord clamping, since current guidance positions cord management as an initial consideration alongside, rather than strictly before, resuscitative support

C. Withhold all resuscitative efforts until this infant has been fully transferred to the warmer and formally reassessed

D. Administer epinephrine immediately, prior to any attempt at establishing effective ventilation

E. Discontinue resuscitative efforts immediately, given this infant's extremely preterm gestational age and initial presentation

Answer: B. Current guidance positions cord management as an initial consideration alongside, not strictly before, resuscitative support — beginning initial steps and ventilation while genuinely deferring clamping where equipment allows.

This vignette directly tests this book's own established resuscitation content: deferred cord clamping represents current, evidence-based practice where the necessary equipment and personnel are genuinely available, and this same practice can genuinely occur alongside, rather than strictly before, initial resuscitative steps.

This infant's own presentation, limp, apnoeic, and bradycardic, directly warrants prompt initial steps and positive pressure ventilation as needed, this same, prompt intervention not requiring this infant to first be fully transferred and cord-clamped before any assessment or support genuinely begins.

This reflects this book's own repeated theme that correctly, safely resuscitating a genuinely critically ill infant requires actively integrating multiple, evidence-based practices together, rather than treating cord management and ventilatory support as sequential, mutually exclusive steps.

Why the other options are wrong

A. Immediate clamping before any assessment does not reflect current, evidence-based, integrated practice.

C. Resuscitative efforts should genuinely begin promptly, not be withheld until full transfer and reassessment.

D. Epinephrine is reserved for continued bradycardia despite effective ventilation and compressions, not as an immediate first step.

E. This gestational age and initial presentation alone do not represent an indication to discontinue resuscitative efforts.

Board Alert Current guidance positions cord management as an initial consideration alongside, not strictly before, resuscitative support — deferred clamping can occur while initial steps and ventilation genuinely proceed.

Question 2

A 33-week gestation infant is delivered by elective caesarean section without labour. At 2 hours of life, this infant demonstrates mild tachypnoea and a chest radiograph shows a streaky, perihilar pattern with fluid visible in the interlobar fissures. Which of the following best distinguishes this presentation from surfactant-deficient respiratory distress syndrome?

A. No genuine, meaningful distinction exists between these two specific conditions of any kind

B. This presentation's own specific radiographic pattern, delivery mode without labour, and typically self-limited course within 24 to 72 hours together are more consistent with transient tachypnoea of the newborn, genuinely distinct from the diffuse, fine granular pattern and air bronchograms characteristic of surfactant deficiency

C. This presentation is more consistent with surfactant-deficient respiratory distress syndrome, given this infant's gestational age alone

D. Delivery mode carries no genuine relevance to distinguishing between these two specific conditions

E. This specific radiographic pattern carries no genuine, diagnostic significance in distinguishing between these two conditions

Answer: B. **This presentation's specific radiographic pattern, delivery without labour, and typically self-limited course are more consistent with transient tachypnoea of the newborn, genuinely distinct from surfactant deficiency's diffuse, granular pattern with air bronchograms.**

This vignette directly tests correctly distinguishing between two, genuinely similar-appearing respiratory presentations: transient tachypnoea of the newborn's own characteristic streaky, perihilar pattern with fluid in the interlobar fissures is genuinely distinct from respiratory distress syndrome's own diffuse, fine granular pattern with air bronchograms.

This infant's own delivery via caesarean section without labour directly connects to this book's established physiology content regarding catecholamine-mediated active fetal lung fluid clearance, normally significantly driven by the physiological stress of active labour, this infant's own genuine absence of this same stress directly elevating risk for delayed fluid clearance specifically.

This same presentation's own typically self-limited, favourable course within 24 to 72 hours, without specific surfactant intervention, further distinguishes this diagnosis from surfactant deficiency, reinforcing this book's repeated theme that correctly, precisely distinguishing between two connected, similar-appearing conditions directly informs appropriate, targeted management.

Why the other options are wrong

A. A genuine, meaningful, distinguishing pattern exists between these two conditions, as detailed in the correct answer.

C. This presentation's specific pattern and course are more consistent with transient tachypnoea, not surfactant deficiency.

D. Delivery mode carries direct, mechanistic relevance to distinguishing these two conditions, as detailed in the correct answer.

E. This specific pattern carries direct, diagnostic significance in distinguishing these two conditions.

Board Alert Transient tachypnoea of the newborn: streaky, perihilar pattern with interlobar fissure fluid, delivery without labour, typically self-limited within 24–72 hours — genuinely distinct from surfactant-deficient RDS.

Question 3

A 28-week gestation infant on day 2 of life has a blood gas showing pH 7.19, PCO2 78 mmHg, and a normal bicarbonate for gestational age. The infant is stable on conventional ventilation with a reasonable oxygen requirement. Which of the following best reflects the correct, current approach to this specific finding?

A. Immediate ventilator escalation is mandatory given this specific PCO2, regardless of clinical stability or pH

B. This finding falls within a pH-controlled permissive hypercapnia range shown in current trial evidence to increase ventilator-free days without significant differences in bronchopulmonary dysplasia or neurodevelopmental harm, supporting continued, careful monitoring in this clinically stable infant rather than reflexive escalation

C. This finding reflects a primary metabolic disturbance requiring bicarbonate correction

D. Clinical stability carries no genuine relevance to correctly interpreting this specific blood gas finding

E. No genuinely current evidence exists regarding an upper carbon dioxide threshold in this specific population

Answer: B. **This finding falls within a pH-controlled permissive hypercapnia range shown to increase ventilator-free days without significant BPD or neurodevelopmental harm, supporting continued monitoring in this clinically stable infant rather than reflexive escalation.**

This vignette directly tests this book's own established acid-base content: the elevated PCO2 with normal bicarbonate reflects a primary respiratory, rather than metabolic, disturbance, and this specific combination falls within the higher, pH-controlled permissive hypercapnia target range established by a genuinely current randomised trial.

This same trial found this higher target range associated with increased ventilator-free days during the 28 days following randomisation, without significant differences in bronchopulmonary dysplasia or evidence of neurodevelopmental harm, directly supporting continued, careful monitoring rather than reflexive escalation in this clinically stable infant.

This reflects this book's own repeated theme of honest evidence treatment: the genuinely current, honestly acknowledged absence of a formally established upper carbon dioxide safety limit supports individualised, careful clinical judgment integrating this infant's own overall stability, rather than a rigid, universal threshold.

Why the other options are wrong

A. This specific PCO2 falls within an evidence-supported target range in this stable infant; immediate escalation is not mandatory.

C. This finding reflects a primary respiratory, not metabolic, disturbance; bicarbonate correction is not indicated.

D. This infant's own clinical stability carries direct, essential relevance to correctly interpreting this finding.

E. Genuinely current trial evidence exists, as detailed in the correct answer, though a formal upper limit remains honestly unestablished.

Board Alert A genuinely current trial found a higher, pH-controlled permissive hypercapnia target associated with increased ventilator-free days, without significant BPD difference or neurodevelopmental harm.

Question 4

A 26-week gestation infant on day 2 of life develops significant hypotension. The clinical team notes this infant's myocardium demonstrates reduced myofibrillar content relative to a term infant's myocardium. Which of the following best explains why this infant's cardiac output remains more dependent on heart rate than on increased preload?

A. This infant's myocardium demonstrates an identical, mature Frank-Starling reserve to a term infant's myocardium

B. Reduced myofibrillar content directly limits this immature myocardium's own capacity to generate increased contractile force in response to increased ventricular filling, meaning this same myocardium relies more heavily on heart rate, through the force-frequency relationship, to maintain adequate cardiac output

C. Heart rate carries no genuine relationship to cardiac output in this specific population

D. This infant's cardiac output is entirely independent of preload, afterload, and heart rate alike at this gestational age

E. This finding carries no genuine, mechanistic explanation of any kind, reflecting an isolated, unconnected observation

Answer: B. **Reduced myofibrillar content directly limits the immature myocardium's capacity to generate increased contractile force with increased filling, meaning this myocardium relies more heavily on heart rate, through the force-frequency relationship, to maintain cardiac output.**

This vignette directly tests this book's own three-part myocardial immaturity framework: reduced myofibrillar content structurally explains a genuinely limited Frank-Starling reserve, meaning this same, immature myocardium cannot generate increased contractile force in response to increased ventricular filling as effectively as a mature, term myocardium.

This same, structural limitation directly explains this immature myocardium's own genuinely elevated, important reliance on heart rate, through the force-frequency relationship, to maintain adequate cardiac output, this same mechanism directly connecting to correctly, safely managing significant hypotension in this exact population.

This reflects this book's own repeated theme that correctly, precisely understanding a specific, structural myocardial limitation directly explains a further, connected physiological compensation, rather than treating this infant's own heart-rate dependence as an isolated, unexplained clinical observation.

Why the other options are wrong

A. This infant's myocardium demonstrates a genuinely limited, not identical, Frank-Starling reserve compared with a term infant.

C. A direct, mechanistic relationship exists between heart rate and cardiac output in this population, as detailed in the correct answer.

D. Cardiac output remains genuinely dependent on all three of these parameters, though the relative contribution of each genuinely differs.

E. A direct, mechanistic explanation exists for this finding, as detailed in the correct answer.

> **Board Alert** Reduced myofibrillar content limits the immature myocardium's Frank-Starling reserve, explaining its elevated reliance on heart rate, through the force-frequency relationship, to maintain adequate cardiac output.

Question 5

A 25-week gestation infant is receiving caffeine citrate for apnoea of prematurity. The clinical team is reviewing dosing given genuinely current pharmacokinetic modelling. Which of the following best reflects the correct, current understanding of this specific medication's dosing considerations?

A. The same, uniform weight-based dosing currently applied to every neonate fully, adequately accounts for differing renal function and gestational-age-specific metabolism

B. Genuinely current pharmacokinetic modelling has shown that the same, uniform weight-based dosing currently applied to every neonate does not account for differing renal function or gestational-age-specific metabolism, supporting individualised dosing consideration, particularly given this medication's own genuinely current, separately identified association with acute kidney injury risk

C. This medication's own dosing carries no genuine relationship to this infant's own gestational age of any kind

D. Renal function carries no genuine relevance to correctly dosing this specific medication

E. This medication should genuinely, immediately be discontinued in every infant, given this genuinely current safety signal

> **Answer: B. Genuinely current pharmacokinetic modelling shows uniform, weight-based caffeine dosing does not account for differing renal function or gestational-age-specific metabolism, supporting individualised dosing given this medication's separately identified acute kidney injury association.**
>
> This vignette directly tests this book's own genuinely current, connected pharmacology content: genuinely current pharmacokinetic modelling has shown that the same, uniform weight-based dosing currently applied to every neonate does not account for differing renal function or gestational-age-specific metabolism.

This same finding directly connects to this book's own separately established, genuinely current safety signal linking early caffeine citrate administration to acute kidney injury risk, together supporting active, individualised dosing consideration rather than a single, uniform approach applied without regard to this infant's own specific, connected renal and gestational-age status.

This reflects this book's own repeated theme that a single medication can carry both genuine, established benefit and a genuine, current safety signal simultaneously, requiring active, individualised clinical judgment rather than either uncritical, uniform dosing or reflexive, complete discontinuation.

Why the other options are wrong

A. Current, uniform dosing does not yet adequately account for these factors, as detailed in the correct answer.

C. A direct, established relationship exists between this medication's dosing and gestational age, as detailed in the correct answer.

D. Renal function carries direct, essential relevance to correctly dosing this medication, as detailed in the correct answer.

E. Individualised dosing, not reflexive, complete discontinuation, represents the correct, current approach.

Board Alert Genuinely current pharmacokinetic modelling shows uniform caffeine dosing fails to account for renal function or gestational-age-specific metabolism, supporting individualised dosing given the separate, associated acute kidney injury risk.

Mock Exam 3 — Section A: Foundations | Universal Task 2: Epidemiology and Risk Assessment

Question 6

A 27-week gestation infant develops a grade II intraventricular haemorrhage on day 4 of life. A review of this infant's own blood gases reveals a significant metabolic acidosis on day 1, but normal acid-base status thereafter. Which of the following best reflects the correct, connected interpretation of this earlier finding?

A. This earlier finding carries no genuine, established relationship to this infant's own subsequent haemorrhage of any kind

B. Genuinely current research has specifically demonstrated that metabolic acidosis, rather than hypocapnia or hypercapnia specifically, occurring within the first 72 hours of life carries a specific, established association with significant intraventricular haemorrhage, directly connecting this earlier, day 1 finding to this infant's own subsequent diagnosis

C. Only hypercapnia, not metabolic acidosis, carries any established relationship to intraventricular haemorrhage risk

D. This specific connection represents an isolated, uncommon finding with no genuine, current research basis of any kind

E. This infant's day 1 finding should have been entirely disregarded once acid-base status subsequently normalised

Answer: B. Genuinely current research demonstrates that metabolic acidosis specifically, occurring within the first 72 hours of life, carries an established association with significant intraventricular haemorrhage — directly connecting this earlier, day 1 finding to this infant's diagnosis.

This vignette directly tests a genuinely important, current distinction this book establishes: it is specifically metabolic acidosis, rather than hypocapnia or hypercapnia, occurring within the first 72 hours of life that carries the established, specific association with significant intraventricular haemorrhage.

This means this infant's own day 1 metabolic acidosis, even though acid-base status subsequently, genuinely normalised, remains directly, connectedly relevant to correctly, retrospectively understanding this same infant's own subsequent haemorrhage, reinforcing this book's repeated theme that a specific, earlier laboratory finding can carry genuine, connected relevance to a later, more serious diagnosis.

This reflects this book's own repeated theme that correctly, completely reviewing a given infant's own clinical course requires actively considering earlier, connected findings, rather than assuming a subsequently normalised value entirely negates that earlier finding's own genuine, diagnostic relevance.

Why the other options are wrong

A. A direct, established relationship exists between this earlier finding and this infant's outcome, as detailed in the correct answer.

C. This reverses the correct relationship; metabolic acidosis, not hypercapnia specifically, carries this specific, established association.

D. This specific connection has direct, genuine basis in current, published research.

E. This earlier finding retains genuine, connected relevance despite subsequent normalisation, as detailed in the correct answer.

Board Alert Metabolic acidosis, specifically, occurring within the first 72 hours of life carries an established, current association with significant intraventricular haemorrhage, regardless of subsequent normalisation.

Question 7

A 22-week gestation fetus is diagnosed with a significant, isolated, life-limiting anomaly. The family expresses interest in perinatal palliative care but also asks whether choosing this pathway means 'giving up' on their baby. Which of the following best reflects the correct, compassionate response to this specific concern?

A. This family's own specific concern should genuinely be dismissed without any further, active, clarifying discussion

B. This family should be reassured that perinatal palliative care represents a genuinely coordinated care strategy directly focused on maximising quality of life and genuine comfort, one option among a genuinely complete, legitimate spectrum, rather than an abandonment of active, compassionate care for their baby

C. This family should genuinely be told that choosing this pathway does, in fact, represent giving up on their baby

D. This family's own specific concern carries no genuine relevance to correctly, compassionately responding to this question

E. This specific pathway should genuinely never be discussed as a legitimate, complete option in any circumstance

Answer: B. This family should be reassured that perinatal palliative care is a genuinely coordinated care strategy focused on maximising quality of life and comfort — one legitimate option among a complete spectrum, not an abandonment of active, compassionate care.

This vignette directly tests this book's own foundational ethics content:

perinatal palliative care, a genuinely coordinated care strategy directly focused on maximising quality of life and genuine comfort for an infant with a life-limiting condition, represents one, specific option along a genuinely broader, legitimate spectrum of care.

This same, genuine reassurance directly addresses this family's own honest, common concern, reinforcing this book's own repeated theme that offering perinatal palliative care should genuinely be seen as an opportunity to further, rather than limit, a family's own genuine autonomy and beneficent, complete care, never representing abandonment.

This reflects this book's own repeated, compassionate communication principle: correctly, honestly addressing a family's own genuine, common misconception directly requires active, clear, and reassuring clarification, rather than dismissal or, worse, confirmation of this same, inaccurate concern.

Why the other options are wrong

A. This concern deserves active, clarifying discussion, not dismissal, as detailed in the correct answer.

C. This pathway does not represent giving up; it represents genuinely coordinated, active, compassionate care.

D. This family's own concern carries direct, essential relevance to correctly, compassionately responding.

E. This pathway represents a genuinely legitimate, complete option that should be discussed, as detailed in the correct answer.

Board Alert Perinatal palliative care is a genuinely coordinated care strategy focused on maximising quality of life and comfort — a legitimate option, never an abandonment of active, compassionate care.

Question 8

A term infant presents with significant respiratory distress, hypotonia, and is subsequently found to have significant hepatomegaly and cardiomegaly. Rapid genome sequencing returns within 30 hours, confirming Pompe disease. Which of the following best reflects the most important, immediate clinical implication of this specific, rapid diagnosis?

A. This diagnosis carries no genuine, specific treatment implication of any kind

B. This rapid, correct diagnosis directly enables early initiation of enzyme replacement therapy, with genuine, significant potential to improve this infant's own eventual outcome, illustrating rapid genomic diagnosis's direct, practical value when a targeted therapy genuinely exists

C. This diagnosis should prompt immediate discontinuation of all supportive respiratory and cardiac care

D. This infant's presentation is entirely unrelated to this newly identified genetic diagnosis

E. Rapid genome sequencing carries no genuine advantage over traditional, sequential genetic testing in this specific circumstance

Answer: B. **This rapid, correct diagnosis directly enables early enzyme replacement therapy, genuinely improving this infant's outcome — illustrating rapid genomic diagnosis's direct, practical value precisely when a targeted therapy exists.**

This vignette directly tests this book's own genuinely important, moving case example: rapid genome sequencing achieving diagnostic turnaround within 24 to 72 hours, here specifically identifying Pompe disease from a presentation of hypotonia, respiratory distress, hepatomegaly, and cardiomegaly.

This diagnosis's own clinical significance lies specifically in its direct connection to available, targeted treatment: enzyme replacement therapy for this specific, genuinely serious lysosomal storage disorder directly benefits from early initiation, making rapid diagnosis genuinely, clinically consequential.

This illustrates this book's own repeated theme that a genuinely rapid, correct genetic diagnosis can directly translate into life-changing treatment specifically when a targeted therapy genuinely exists for the condition identified.

Why the other options are wrong

A. This diagnosis carries a direct, significant treatment implication, as detailed in the correct answer.

C. This condition has a specific, genuine treatment option; supportive care should continue alongside, not be discontinued.

D. This infant's presentation is directly, mechanistically explained by this newly identified diagnosis.

E. Rapid sequencing's genuinely faster turnaround carries direct, practical advantage in this time-sensitive circumstance.

Board Alert Rapid genome sequencing's clinical value is most dramatic when it identifies a treatable condition — Pompe disease directly connects rapid diagnosis to early, life-changing enzyme replacement therapy.

Question 9

A 24-week gestation infant is delivered and immediately dried and wrapped, then placed under a radiant warmer without a polyethylene bag or warming mattress at a smaller, referring facility genuinely lacking this specific equipment. Admission temperature is 34.8°C. Which of the following best reflects the correct, honest interpretation of this specific circumstance?

A. This finding reflects a normal, expected outcome requiring no further, active consideration of any kind

B. This finding should prompt active recognition that this facility's own specific, available equipment did not include the combined, multimodal thermal approach this book establishes as targeting multiple, distinct mechanisms of heat loss together, supporting active advocacy for improved equipment access alongside careful, ongoing thermal management

C. Drying and radiant warming alone provide an entirely equivalent thermal approach to the full, combined, multimodal strategy

D. This infant's own extremely preterm gestational age carries no genuine relevance to this specific thermal outcome

E. This specific facility's own equipment limitations carry no genuine relevance to this outcome of any kind

Answer: B. This finding should prompt recognition that this facility's available equipment did not include the combined, multimodal thermal approach targeting multiple distinct heat-loss mechanisms together — supporting advocacy for improved equipment access alongside careful, ongoing management.

This vignette directly tests this book's own established thermal physiology content: the combined, multimodal thermal approach — polyethylene wrapping without drying for evaporative loss, warmed environment for convective loss, and a warming mattress for conductive loss — targets multiple, distinct mechanisms of heat loss simultaneously.

This infant's own significant hypothermia, occurring at a facility genuinely lacking this same, full, combined approach, directly illustrates why this multimodal strategy carries genuine, particular importance for this extremely preterm population, this population's own genuinely elevated surface-area-to-body-mass ratio and reduced subcutaneous insulation making thermal vulnerability genuinely significant.

This reflects this book's own repeated, systems-level theme, connecting directly to this book's own care systems content: correctly, safely caring for this population requires active attention not only to individual clinical technique, but to this facility's own broader, connected equipment and resource access.

Why the other options are wrong

A. This finding warrants active consideration and systems-level attention, not assumption of a normal, expected outcome.

C. This more limited approach does not provide an entirely equivalent thermal effect compared with the full, combined strategy.

D. This infant's own gestational age carries direct, genuine relevance to this thermal outcome, as detailed in the correct answer.

E. This facility's own equipment limitations carry direct, genuine relevance to this outcome.

Board Alert The combined, multimodal thermal approach targets multiple, distinct mechanisms of heat loss simultaneously; equipment limitations at a given facility carry direct, systems-level relevance to thermal outcomes.

Mock Exam 3 — Section B: Organ Systems | Universal Task 3: Diagnosis, Testing and Monitoring

Question 10

A 27-week gestation infant is 3 weeks old and remains on continuous positive airway pressure with an oxygen requirement of 35 per cent. The clinical team is reviewing this infant's own connected risk factors for evolving bronchopulmonary dysplasia. Which of the following combined risk factors, if present, would most directly reflect this book's own established, bidirectional risk framework?

A. A history of significant hypercapnia alone, with no genuine relevance from any other, connected acid-base parameter

B. A history of both significant hypocapnia occurring before surfactant therapy and early metabolic acidosis, since each has been independently associated with increased risk, reflecting a genuinely bidirectional and multifactorial risk profile requiring active avoidance of extremes in both directions

C. This infant's own gestational age carries no genuine relevance to this specific risk profile

D. No genuinely established, connected risk factor exists for evolving bronchopulmonary dysplasia of any kind

E. Ventilator strategy carries no genuine relationship to this specific diagnosis's own risk profile

Answer: B. A history of both significant hypocapnia before surfactant therapy and early metabolic acidosis, each independently associated with increased risk, reflects a genuinely bidirectional, multifactorial risk profile requiring avoidance of extremes in both directions.

This vignette directly tests this book's own repeated, bidirectional risk theme for bronchopulmonary dysplasia: significant hypocapnia occurring before surfactant therapy has itself been associated with increased risk, while separately, genuinely current research has demonstrated an association between early metabolic acidosis and this same diagnosis.

This reflects this book's own repeated theme that safe, correctly calibrated ventilator and acid-base management requires actively avoiding excess in either direction — neither excessive hypocapnia nor significant metabolic acidosis represents a genuinely safe extreme, each independently carrying connected, elevated risk.

This connected, multifactorial risk profile directly reinforces why this book has emphasised structured, careful acid-base and ventilator management throughout its own foundational content, rather than focusing on carbon dioxide management alone in isolation from this infant's own broader, connected metabolic status.

Why the other options are wrong

A. Both hypocapnia and metabolic acidosis, not hypercapnia alone, carry established, connected relationships to this diagnosis.

C. This infant's own gestational age carries direct, established relevance to this diagnosis's own risk profile.

D. Specific, established, connected risk factors exist, as detailed in the correct answer.

E. A direct, established relationship exists between ventilation strategy and this specific diagnosis's own risk.

Board Alert Bronchopulmonary dysplasia risk is genuinely bidirectional and multifactorial: significant hypocapnia before surfactant therapy and early metabolic acidosis have each been independently associated with increased risk.

Question 11

A 26-week gestation infant develops significant abdominal distension on day 15 of life. Abdominal radiography demonstrates pneumatosis intestinalis. Over the following 6 hours, this infant develops worsening lactic acidosis and a new, free intraperitoneal air collection on repeat imaging. Which of the following represents the correct, immediate next step?

A. Continued medical management alone, without any active, further surgical consideration, since pneumatosis intestinalis alone was the only finding initially present

B. This infant should proceed urgently to surgical intervention, since this new finding of pneumoperitoneum represents the sole absolute indication for immediate surgery in necrotising enterocolitis

C. This infant's worsening lactic acidosis alone, without any further, connected finding, represents sufficient indication for surgery

D. Repeat imaging carries no genuine relevance to this infant's own evolving surgical decision-making

E. This infant should be observed for a further, extended period before any active, surgical reconsideration

Answer: B. This infant should proceed urgently to surgery, since this new finding of pneumoperitoneum on repeat imaging represents the sole absolute indication for immediate surgical intervention in necrotising enterocolitis.

This vignette directly tests this book's own foundational surgical principle applied to an evolving, dynamic clinical picture: while pneumatosis intestinalis alone did not initially represent an absolute surgical indication, this infant's own subsequent, new pneumoperitoneum on repeat imaging directly represents this single, unambiguous, absolute indication for immediate surgery.

This infant's own worsening lactic acidosis, while genuinely important and connected, reflects one of several genuinely important, but non-absolute, indicators requiring integrated, dynamic clinical assessment, whereas the new pneumoperitoneum finding stands apart, unambiguous and immediately actionable.

This reflects this book's own repeated theme that this genuinely uncertain surgical decision-making landscape requires active, dynamic, ongoing reassessment, since a given infant's own clinical picture, and this same infant's own specific, appropriate management, can genuinely, rapidly evolve over a relatively short period of time.

Why the other options are wrong

A. This new, connected finding directly changes this infant's own management, warranting urgent surgical intervention.

C. This finding alone, without the specific pneumoperitoneum finding, does not represent this same, single absolute indication.

D. Repeat imaging carries direct, essential relevance to this infant's own evolving decision-making, as detailed in the correct answer.

E. This new, absolute surgical indication warrants urgent action, not further, extended observation.

Board Alert Pneumoperitoneum, even when it develops after an initial presentation of pneumatosis alone, represents the sole absolute indication for immediate surgery in necrotising enterocolitis, warranting urgent reassessment.

Mock Exam 3 — Section B: Organ Systems | Universal Task 3: Diagnosis, Testing and Monitoring

Question 12

A term infant develops significant cyanosis at 12 hours of life that improves only minimally with 100 per cent supplemental oxygen. A hyperoxia test confirms a PaO2 that remains below 100 mmHg. Which of the following best reflects the correct, immediate diagnostic priority?

A. This presentation should be managed exclusively as primary pulmonary disease, without any further, active cardiac evaluation

B. This infant's own limited response to supplemental oxygen should prompt urgent echocardiographic evaluation for significant, structural congenital heart disease, given this specific finding's own established relevance to distinguishing cardiac from pulmonary causes of cyanosis

C. A hyperoxia test carries no genuine, diagnostic utility in evaluating significant, neonatal cyanosis

D. This infant's own specific response to supplemental oxygen carries no genuine, diagnostic significance of any kind

E. This presentation requires no further, active or urgent evaluation of any kind

Answer: B. This infant's limited response to supplemental oxygen should prompt urgent echocardiographic evaluation for significant, structural congenital heart disease, given this finding's established relevance to distinguishing cardiac from pulmonary causes of cyanosis.

This vignette directly tests the classic, foundational hyperoxia test: a genuinely limited rise in PaO2 despite 100 per cent supplemental oxygen directly reflects a fixed, structural right-to-left shunt characteristic of significant congenital heart disease, genuinely distinct from primary pulmonary disease, which typically demonstrates a considerably more significant rise with supplemental oxygen.

This specific, connected finding directly supports urgent echocardiographic evaluation, since correctly, rapidly distinguishing between these two, genuinely different specific categories of cyanosis directly informs the appropriate, urgent, and potentially life-saving management this infant genuinely requires.

This reflects this book's own repeated theme that correctly, precisely interpreting a specific, connected diagnostic test directly changes the appropriate, immediate management approach, rather than assuming every case of significant, neonatal cyanosis reflects an identical, underlying cause.

Why the other options are wrong

A. This specific finding suggests a cardiac, not exclusively pulmonary, cause, warranting active cardiac evaluation.

C. This specific test carries direct, established diagnostic utility, as detailed in the correct answer.

D. This specific response carries direct, diagnostic significance in this specific clinical context.

E. This presentation warrants urgent, active evaluation, as detailed in the correct answer.

Board Alert A hyperoxia test showing limited PaO2 rise despite 100 per cent supplemental oxygen suggests a fixed, structural right-to-left cardiac shunt, warranting urgent echocardiographic evaluation.

Question 13

A 28-week gestation infant is 3 weeks old and being advanced on enteral feeds using fortified maternal expressed milk. The clinical team notes a rising alkaline phosphatase and mild osteopenia on a routine radiograph obtained for another indication. Which of the following best reflects the correct, connected understanding of this specific finding?

- **A.** This finding carries no genuine, connected relationship to this infant's own nutritional status of any kind
- **B.** This finding is consistent with metabolic bone disease of prematurity, directly connecting to this population's own genuinely elevated calcium and phosphorus requirements, supporting active review of this infant's own current fortification adequacy
- **C.** This finding requires no further, active nutritional review or connected management of any kind
- **D.** Alkaline phosphatase elevation in this specific context carries no genuine, diagnostic significance of any kind
- **E.** This infant's own gestational age carries no genuine relevance to this specific finding

Answer: B. This finding is consistent with metabolic bone disease of prematurity, connecting to this population's genuinely elevated calcium and phosphorus requirements, supporting active review of current fortification adequacy.

This vignette directly tests this book's own established nutrition content: this population's own genuinely elevated calcium and phosphorus requirements directly connect to this same population's own genuine, elevated risk of metabolic bone disease of prematurity, this specific finding — elevated alkaline phosphatase with radiographic osteopenia — representing this condition's own characteristic, connected presentation.

This same finding directly supports active review of this infant's own current fortification adequacy, since correctly, adequately meeting these same, elevated mineral requirements through appropriate, sufficient fortification represents the correct, connected management approach.

This reflects this book's own repeated theme that correctly, individually tailoring nutritional support to this population's own genuinely distinctive requirements directly supports this same population's own genuine, connected bone health, requiring active, ongoing nutritional attention and periodic reassessment throughout this infant's own hospitalisation.

Why the other options are wrong

A. A direct, established relationship exists between this finding and nutritional status, as detailed in the correct answer.

C. Active nutritional review and connected management are genuinely warranted for this specific finding.

D. This specific marker carries direct, diagnostic significance in this connected presentation.

E. This infant's own gestational age carries direct, genuine relevance to this specific finding's own risk profile.

Board Alert Elevated alkaline phosphatase with radiographic osteopenia is consistent with metabolic bone disease of prematurity, supporting active review of fortification adequacy given elevated calcium and phosphorus requirements.

Mock Exam 3 — Section B: Organ Systems | Universal Task 3: Diagnosis, Testing and Monitoring

Question 14

A term infant develops significant respiratory distress at birth and is noted to have a small, receding chin, cleft palate, and significant, positional airway obstruction. Genetic testing later confirms an isolated, non-syndromic presentation. Which of the following best reflects the correct, connected management priority once this infant's airway has been positionally stabilised?

A. No further, active airway management planning is genuinely required once initial, positional stabilisation has been achieved

B. Active, ongoing airway assessment and planning remain genuinely important, since this infant's own connected obstruction can persist or worsen, potentially requiring further, definitive intervention beyond positioning alone as this infant continues to grow and develop

C. This infant's own confirmed, isolated presentation eliminates any further, genuine need for active airway monitoring

D. Cleft palate carries no genuine, connected relevance to this infant's own ongoing airway management

E. This infant requires no further, active or structured, connected follow-up of any kind

Answer: B. **Active, ongoing airway assessment and planning remain genuinely important, since this infant's connected obstruction can persist or worsen, potentially requiring further, definitive intervention beyond positioning alone as this infant continues to grow.**

This vignette directly tests this book's own established Pierre Robin sequence content, extended to this infant's own longer-term, connected management: while prone positioning often provides genuine, immediate improvement in the acute, neonatal period, this same, connected obstruction can genuinely persist or evolve as this infant continues to grow and develop.

Active, ongoing airway assessment therefore remains genuinely important, since further, definitive intervention, potentially including specific surgical management, may genuinely become necessary beyond positioning alone, this same, structured follow-up directly reflecting this book's own repeated theme regarding ongoing, connected clinical vigilance rather than a single, static assessment.

This reflects this book's own repeated theme that correctly, safely managing a specific, connected anatomical sequence requires active attention extending well beyond this infant's own immediate, initial stabilisation alone, into this same infant's own longer-term, evolving clinical course.

Why the other options are wrong

A. Active, ongoing airway planning remains genuinely important, as detailed in the correct answer, not concluding at initial stabilisation.

C. This confirmed, isolated presentation does not eliminate the genuine need for ongoing airway monitoring.

D. This specific finding carries direct, connected relevance to this infant's own ongoing airway management.

E. Active, structured, connected follow-up is genuinely warranted for this specific presentation.

Board Alert Following initial positional stabilisation in Pierre Robin sequence, active, ongoing airway assessment remains genuinely important, since obstruction can persist or worsen as this infant continues to grow.

Question 15

A term infant born to a mother with poorly controlled Graves disease develops significant tachycardia and irritability in the first week of life. The clinical team is discussing this infant's own connected cardiovascular risk. Which of the following represents the most important, active management consideration?

- **A.** No specific, active cardiovascular monitoring is genuinely warranted in this specific circumstance
- **B.** Active, structured monitoring for significant cardiovascular complication, including tachyarrhythmia and, in severe cases, cardiac failure, together with specific treatment where genuinely indicated, represents the correct, appropriate approach, given this condition's own genuine, connected potential for significant complication
- **C.** This infant's presentation carries no genuine, connected relationship to any specific cardiovascular risk of any kind
- **D.** This presentation should genuinely be expected to spontaneously, safely resolve without any active clinical attention of any kind
- **E.** Maternal thyroid antibody status carries no genuine relevance to this infant's own cardiovascular risk

Answer: B. Active, structured monitoring for significant cardiovascular complication, including tachyarrhythmia and cardiac failure, together with specific treatment where indicated, represents the correct approach, given this condition's genuine potential for significant complication.

This vignette directly tests this book's own established endocrine content regarding neonatal Graves disease: maternal thyroid-stimulating immunoglobulins directly cross the placenta and stimulate this infant's own thyroid gland, producing a transient, but genuinely significant, hyperthyroid state.

This condition carries genuine, potential significance for significant cardiovascular complication, including tachyarrhythmia and, in severe cases, cardiac failure, meaning active, structured monitoring and, where genuinely indicated, specific treatment represent the correct, appropriate approach.

This reflects this book's own repeated theme that correctly, safely managing this specific, transient but genuinely significant condition requires active clinical attention, rather than assuming this presentation will spontaneously, safely resolve without any active, structured, connected clinical vigilance.

Why the other options are wrong

A. Active, structured monitoring is genuinely warranted, given this condition's own genuine, connected complication risk.

C. This presentation carries a direct, well-established, connected relationship to this specific cardiovascular risk.

D. Active clinical attention remains genuinely warranted, not passive assumption of spontaneous, safe resolution.

E. Maternal antibody status carries direct, mechanistic relevance to this infant's own presentation and risk.

Board Alert Neonatal Graves disease carries genuine potential for significant cardiovascular complication, including tachyarrhythmia and cardiac failure, requiring active, structured monitoring and treatment where indicated.

Mock Exam 3 — Section B: Organ Systems | Universal Task 3: Diagnosis, Testing and Monitoring

Question 16

A 29-week gestation infant develops a new, significant heart murmur on day 4 of life, together with bounding pulses and a widened pulse pressure. This infant had received surfactant on day 1 with substantial, subsequent improvement in oxygenation. Which of the following best explains the connected, underlying mechanism linking these two, temporally separated events?

A. These two events are entirely coincidental and mechanistically unrelated to one another

B. The rapid fall in pulmonary vascular resistance following surfactant-mediated improvement in oxygenation has unmasked a haemodynamically significant patent ductus arteriosus, now shunting left-to-right, as pulmonary pressure dropped below systemic pressure

C. This murmur reflects a new, unrelated structural cardiac malformation with no genuine, connected relationship to this infant's own respiratory course

D. Surfactant administration carries no genuine, mechanistic relationship to pulmonary vascular resistance of any kind

E. This presentation requires no further, active cardiovascular evaluation of any kind

Answer: B. **The rapid fall in pulmonary vascular resistance following surfactant-mediated improvement in oxygenation has unmasked a haemodynamically significant, left-to-right shunting patent ductus arteriosus, as pulmonary pressure dropped below systemic pressure.**

This vignette directly tests the connected physiology this book establishes repeatedly: a widened pulse pressure and bounding pulses following respiratory improvement represent the classic, connected presentation of a haemodynamically significant patent ductus arteriosus, not a coincidental, unrelated finding.

The mechanism is directly physiological: as surfactant improves oxygenation and lung compliance, pulmonary vascular resistance falls further, and once pulmonary pressure drops below systemic pressure, ductal flow reverses to left-to-right, unmasking a shunt that may have been clinically silent while pulmonary pressures remained elevated.

This connection between respiratory improvement and ductal unmasking represents exactly the kind of cross-system reasoning this book has modelled throughout — recognising that a single, underlying physiological principle explains an apparently new, but genuinely connected, clinical finding occurring days after the initial, connected intervention.

Why the other options are wrong

A. These events are directly, mechanistically connected, as detailed in the correct answer, not coincidental.

C. This murmur is more consistent with a connected, physiological consequence than an unrelated, new structural malformation.

D. A direct, mechanistic relationship exists between surfactant administration and pulmonary vascular resistance.

E. Active cardiovascular evaluation is genuinely warranted for this specific, new finding.

Board Alert Improved oxygenation after surfactant lowers pulmonary vascular resistance, frequently unmasking a haemodynamically significant PDA days later as pulmonary pressure falls below systemic pressure.

Question 17

A term infant with confirmed group B Streptococcus bacteraemia is being treated with appropriate intravenous antibiotics. Cerebrospinal fluid analysis is normal, without pleocytosis. Which of the following best reflects the correct, connected understanding of this infant's own appropriate treatment duration?

A. This infant requires an identical, extended treatment duration to a confirmed case of meningitis, regardless of this infant's own normal cerebrospinal fluid findings

B. This infant's own normal cerebrospinal fluid findings, confirming an absence of central nervous system involvement, directly inform a genuinely shorter, appropriate treatment duration compared with confirmed meningitis, reflecting this book's own repeated theme that correctly, precisely characterising a given infection's own specific extent directly determines appropriate treatment duration

C. Cerebrospinal fluid findings carry no genuine relevance to correctly determining this infant's own appropriate treatment duration

D. This infant requires no further, active antibiotic treatment given this infant's own normal cerebrospinal fluid findings

E. This infant's own confirmed bacteraemia carries no genuine relationship to this infant's own required treatment duration

Answer: B. **This infant's normal cerebrospinal fluid findings, confirming absence of CNS involvement, directly inform a genuinely shorter, appropriate treatment duration compared with confirmed meningitis, since precisely characterising infection**

extent determines appropriate duration.

This vignette directly tests correctly distinguishing uncomplicated bacteraemia from meningitis, directly extending this book's own established infectious disease content: confirmed, culture-positive bacteraemia without central nervous system involvement, confirmed by normal cerebrospinal fluid findings, carries a genuinely different, appropriate treatment duration compared with confirmed meningitis.

This infant's own normal cerebrospinal fluid findings directly inform a genuinely shorter, appropriate antibiotic treatment duration, reflecting this book's own repeated theme that correctly, precisely characterising a given infection's own specific extent directly determines the appropriate, targeted treatment duration this infant genuinely requires.

This reflects this book's own repeated theme that correctly, completely evaluating a confirmed infection requires active, structured determination of this same infection's own specific extent, rather than applying an identical, uniform treatment duration regardless of confirmed central nervous system involvement or its own genuine absence.

Why the other options are wrong

A. This infant's own confirmed absence of CNS involvement warrants a genuinely shorter, not identical, treatment duration.

C. These findings carry direct, essential relevance to determining appropriate treatment duration, as detailed in the correct answer.

D. Continued, appropriate antibiotic treatment remains genuinely required for this confirmed bacteraemia.

E. A direct, established relationship exists between this bacteraemia and this infant's own required treatment duration.

Board Alert Confirmed bacteraemia without CNS involvement, confirmed by normal cerebrospinal fluid findings, warrants a genuinely shorter, appropriate treatment duration compared with confirmed meningitis.

Mock Exam 3 — Section B: Organ Systems | Universal Task 3: Diagnosis, Testing and Monitoring

Question 18

A term infant develops significant abdominal distension and bilious emesis at 36 hours of life. Upper gastrointestinal contrast study demonstrates a corkscrew pattern with the duodenojejunal junction positioned abnormally to the right of the spine. Which of the following represents the most appropriate, immediate management step?

A. Observation and reassurance alone, since this specific radiographic finding carries no genuine, urgent significance

B. This finding is highly consistent with intestinal malrotation with volvulus, a genuinely emergent, time-critical surgical condition, requiring immediate surgical consultation and intervention given the genuine risk of catastrophic, extensive bowel loss from compromised mesenteric blood supply

C. This presentation should be managed exclusively with nasogastric decompression alone, without any further, active surgical evaluation

D. This specific radiographic pattern carries no genuine, diagnostic significance in this specific clinical context

E. This infant should genuinely be observed for several additional days before any active, surgical reconsideration

Answer: B. **This corkscrew pattern with an abnormally positioned duodenojejunal junction is highly consistent with intestinal malrotation with volvulus, a genuinely emergent, time-critical surgical condition requiring immediate consultation and intervention.**

This vignette presents the classic, characteristic radiographic finding for intestinal malrotation with volvulus: a corkscrew pattern on upper gastrointestinal contrast study together with an abnormally positioned duodenojejunal junction directly reflects abnormal intestinal rotation with a narrow mesenteric pedicle around which the bowel has twisted.

This specific twisting can directly, rapidly compromise the entire mesenteric blood supply, threatening genuinely catastrophic, extensive bowel loss within a genuinely narrow, time-critical window, meaning this presentation demands immediate, urgent surgical consultation and intervention rather than observation or nasogastric decompression alone.

This reflects this book's own repeated, urgent theme regarding bilious emesis and this specific, connected condition: correctly, rapidly recognising this specific, characteristic radiographic pattern directly changes the appropriate, immediate management approach, given this presentation's own genuine, catastrophic surgical urgency.

Why the other options are wrong

A. This finding carries genuine, urgent, time-critical significance, not warranting observation and reassurance alone.

C. Immediate surgical evaluation, not nasogastric decompression alone, represents the correct, immediate priority.

D. This specific pattern carries direct, established diagnostic significance in this specific clinical context.

E. This presentation demands immediate, not delayed, surgical evaluation, given its genuine, catastrophic urgency.

Board Alert A corkscrew pattern with an abnormally positioned duodenojejunal junction is highly consistent with intestinal malrotation with volvulus, a genuinely emergent, time-critical surgical condition requiring immediate intervention.

Question 19

A 25-week gestation infant is 4 weeks old and has demonstrated stage 2 retinopathy of prematurity without plus disease on the most recent, structured examination. Which of the following best reflects the correct, current, evidence-based approach to this specific finding?

A. Treatment should genuinely be initiated immediately, regardless of this infant's own specific stage or presence of plus disease

B. Continued, structured, serial ophthalmologic examination on an appropriate, individualised schedule represents the correct, appropriate approach at this specific stage, since this same, ongoing surveillance directly informs the correct, timely treatment decision should genuine progression toward treatment-warranted disease actually occur

C. This infant requires no further, active ophthalmologic surveillance of any kind following this specific examination

D. This infant's own specific stage carries no genuine relevance to correctly determining appropriate management

E. A single, isolated examination at this stage provides an entirely complete, sufficient evaluation with no further follow-up required

Answer: B. Continued, structured, serial examination represents the correct approach at this specific stage, since ongoing

surveillance directly informs the correct, timely treatment decision should genuine progression toward treatment-warranted disease actually occur.

This vignette directly tests this book's own established ophthalmology content: retinopathy of prematurity represents a genuinely dynamic, potentially progressive condition requiring structured, serial examination rather than either immediate treatment at every stage or a single, isolated assessment.

This infant's own current stage 2 findings, without plus disease, do not yet meet established treatment criteria, meaning continued, structured, serial examination on an appropriate, individualised schedule represents the correct, current approach, directly informing the correct, timely treatment decision should genuine progression occur.

This reflects this book's own repeated theme that correctly, safely managing this genuinely dynamic clinical condition requires active, structured, ongoing surveillance, rather than either premature intervention or complete cessation of monitoring at a stage not yet meeting established treatment criteria.

Why the other options are wrong

A. Treatment is reserved for specific, defined criteria not yet met at this stage; immediate treatment is not indicated here.

C. Continued, active surveillance remains genuinely warranted at this stage, given this condition's own potential for progression.

D. This infant's own specific stage carries direct, essential relevance to correctly determining appropriate management.

E. Continued, serial follow-up, not a single, isolated examination, represents the correct, appropriate approach.

Board Alert Stage 2 retinopathy of prematurity without plus disease warrants continued, structured, serial examination rather than immediate treatment, since this condition can genuinely progress toward treatment-warranted disease.

Question 20

A term infant develops significant, progressive direct hyperbilirubinaemia beginning at 2 weeks of life, together with acholic stools. Hepatobiliary scintigraphy shows no evidence of tracer excretion into the bowel after 24 hours. Which of the following best reflects the correct, immediate next step given this infant's own approaching age?

- **A.** Continued observation alone for a further, extended period, since this infant's own current age still provides ample time before any active, surgical consideration
- **B.** Urgent surgical consultation for consideration of Kasai portoenterostomy should be pursued without further delay, given this specific finding's own strong support for biliary atresia and this condition's own genuinely time-sensitive surgical treatment window
- **C.** This specific scintigraphy finding carries no genuine, diagnostic significance in this specific clinical context
- **D.** This presentation should be managed exclusively with continued, structured phototherapy, without any further, active surgical evaluation
- **E.** This infant's own specific age carries no genuine relevance to correctly, urgently planning this infant's own surgical management

Answer: B. Urgent surgical consultation for Kasai portoenterostomy should be pursued without further delay, given this finding's strong support for biliary atresia and this condition's genuinely time-sensitive surgical treatment window.

This vignette directly tests this book's own established, time-sensitive surgical content: absent tracer excretion on hepatobiliary scintigraphy, together with progressive direct hyperbilirubinaemia and acholic stools, strongly supports biliary atresia, this same, connected combination requiring urgent, rather than delayed, evaluation.

This infant's own approaching age directly heightens this specific urgency, since the Kasai portoenterostomy carries genuinely, considerably better outcomes when performed before approximately 8 weeks of age, making prompt surgical consultation and intervention directly, genuinely time-sensitive.

This reflects this book's own repeated theme that correctly, rapidly recognising a specific, connected clinical and diagnostic pattern directly changes the appropriate, immediate management approach, given this specific presentation's own genuine, time-critical surgical urgency.

Why the other options are wrong

- **A.** This infant's own approaching age makes further, extended delay genuinely inappropriate, given this condition's time-sensitive window.

C. This finding carries direct, significant diagnostic significance in this specific clinical context.

D. Urgent surgical evaluation, not phototherapy alone, represents the correct approach for this predominantly direct process.

E. This infant's own age carries direct, urgent relevance to planning surgical management, as detailed in the correct answer.

Board Alert Absent tracer excretion on hepatobiliary scintigraphy, with progressive direct hyperbilirubinaemia and acholic stools, strongly supports biliary atresia — urgent surgical consultation is warranted given the time-sensitive Kasai window.

Question 21

A 31-week gestation infant develops a significant, new-onset seizure on day 5 of life. Glucose, calcium, sodium, and cranial ultrasound are all normal. This infant's mother recalls a similar, unexplained neonatal death in a maternal uncle. Which of the following best reflects the correct, active diagnostic consideration this specific family history should prompt?

A. This family history carries no genuine relevance to correctly evaluating this infant's own seizure of any kind

B. Active consideration of a specific, underlying inborn error of metabolism should genuinely be heightened given this connected family history, with the critical sample principle, correctly timing specific laboratory collection during genuine, active clinical decompensation, carrying direct, particular importance in this specific evaluation

C. This presentation should be managed exclusively as idiopathic seizure, without any further, active diagnostic evaluation

D. Normal, routine metabolic studies and cranial ultrasound entirely exclude any further, active diagnostic consideration

E. This specific family history carries relevance exclusively to this infant's own psychosocial, rather than medical, evaluation

Answer: B. Active consideration of an underlying inborn error of

metabolism should be heightened given this connected family history, with the critical sample principle carrying particular importance in this specific evaluation.

This vignette directly tests this book's own established principle, now reinforced by a genuinely important, connected family history: a genuinely important, broader differential for neonatal seizure includes an inborn error of metabolism, which routine, standard metabolic studies alone do not entirely exclude.

This infant's own connected family history of an unexplained neonatal death directly heightens this same, active diagnostic consideration, reinforcing this book's own repeated theme that correctly, comprehensively evaluating a genuinely concerning presentation requires actively integrating connected family history alongside this infant's own specific, presenting clinical findings.

The critical sample principle, established throughout this book's own endocrine and genetics content, directly extends to this specific circumstance: obtaining specific, relevant laboratory samples at the precise moment of genuine, active clinical decompensation directly provides the most genuinely diagnostic, otherwise fleeting information.

Why the other options are wrong

A. This family history carries direct, genuine relevance to this evaluation, as detailed in the correct answer.

C. This presentation warrants active, specific diagnostic evaluation, not management as idiopathic seizure alone.

D. A normal, routine evaluation does not necessarily, entirely exclude a further, genuinely important diagnostic category.

E. This family history carries direct, genuine medical relevance to this infant's own diagnostic evaluation.

Board Alert A connected family history of unexplained neonatal death should heighten active consideration of an inborn error of metabolism, with the critical sample principle carrying particular importance in this evaluation.

Mock Exam 3 — Section B: Organ Systems | Universal Task 4: Management, Treatment and Prevention

Question 22

A 26-week gestation infant is 2 weeks old and remains on mechanical ventilation. The clinical team is discussing correctly, safely applying sedation for an upcoming, minor procedure. This infant has already received a genuinely prolonged, 6-day continuous fentanyl infusion for a separate indication. Which of the following best reflects the correct, connected consideration this specific circumstance requires?

A. This infant's own prior, prolonged opioid exposure carries no genuine relevance to correctly planning this upcoming procedure's own sedation

B. This infant's own genuinely prolonged, 6-day infusion carries a genuine, significant risk of narcotic withdrawal symptoms upon eventual discontinuation, requiring active, structured attention to both this infant's own procedural sedation needs and this same, connected, gradual weaning consideration

C. This infant's own prior opioid exposure carries no genuine, connected relationship to withdrawal risk of any kind

D. This infant requires no further, active pain or withdrawal assessment of any kind, given this infant's own current, ongoing infusion

E. Infusion duration carries no genuine, meaningful relationship to withdrawal risk of any kind

Answer: B. **This infant's genuinely prolonged, 6-day infusion carries a significant risk of narcotic withdrawal symptoms upon eventual discontinuation, requiring active attention to both procedural sedation needs and gradual weaning consideration together.**

This vignette directly tests this book's own established pharmacology content: neonates genuinely treated with a continuous opioid infusion for a genuinely prolonged duration, established as approximately 5 days or considerably longer, are genuinely, significantly more likely to develop specific narcotic withdrawal symptoms once this infusion is genuinely, eventually discontinued.

This infant's own 6-day infusion duration directly exceeds this specific, practical threshold, meaning correctly, safely managing this infant's own ongoing care requires active, structured attention to both this infant's own procedural sedation needs for the upcoming procedure and this same, connected, eventual, gradual weaning consideration.

This reflects this book's own repeated theme that a specific medication's own genuine, connected risk frequently extends well beyond its own initial administration, requiring active, ongoing clinical attention throughout the entire, genuine duration of treatment and into its own eventual, careful discontinuation.

Why the other options are wrong

A. This prior exposure carries direct, genuine relevance to planning this procedure's sedation, as detailed in the correct answer.

C. A direct, established relationship exists between this exposure and withdrawal risk, as detailed in the correct answer.

D. Active, ongoing pain and withdrawal assessment remains genuinely important throughout this infusion.

E. A direct, established relationship exists between infusion duration and withdrawal risk, as detailed in the correct answer.

Board Alert Neonates receiving a continuous opioid infusion for approximately 5 days or longer are significantly more likely to develop narcotic withdrawal symptoms, requiring active attention to gradual weaning.

Mock Exam 3 — Section B: Organ Systems | Universal Task 3: Diagnosis, Testing and Monitoring

Question 23

A term infant is noted to have significant micrognathia, low-set ears, rocker-bottom feet, and a significant, clenched hand posture with overlapping fingers. Growth parameters are significantly below expected. Which of the following genetic diagnoses is most strongly suggested by this specific, connected combination of findings, and what is the correct, honest approach to family counselling?

A. This combination of findings carries no genuine, connected relationship to any specific genetic diagnosis of any kind

B. This presentation is highly suggestive of trisomy 18, and honest, complete counselling should acknowledge this specific diagnosis's own considerably more severe, connected pattern of anomalies and correspondingly more limited prognosis, together with the full, complete spectrum of reasonable care options

C. This presentation is more consistent with trisomy 21, which typically carries a considerably more severe, connected pattern of findings than described here

D. This specific combination of findings carries an identical, generic counselling approach regardless of this infant's own specific, underlying chromosomal diagnosis

E. This family's own genuine values carry no genuine relevance to this specific counselling conversation

Answer: B. **This presentation is highly suggestive of trisomy 18. Honest counselling should acknowledge this diagnosis's own considerably more severe, connected pattern of anomalies and correspondingly more limited prognosis, together with the full spectrum of options.**

This vignette presents the classic, connected combination for trisomy 18: micrognathia, low-set ears, rocker-bottom feet, and a characteristic clenched hand posture with overlapping fingers together represent this specific trisomy's own characteristic, connected dysmorphic pattern.

This connected reasoning — recognising that a single, underlying chromosomal abnormality directly explains multiple, apparently distinct findings together — represents exactly the kind of mechanism-first, pattern-recognition diagnostic reasoning this book has modelled throughout its own genetics content.

Honest, complete family counselling directly requires acknowledging this specific diagnosis's own considerably more severe, connected pattern of significant major congenital anomalies and correspondingly, genuinely more limited overall prognosis compared with trisomy 21, together with the full, complete spectrum of reasonable care options this family deserves.

Why the other options are wrong

A. A direct, well-established, connected relationship exists between this combination and this specific diagnosis.

C. This presentation is more classically, specifically associated with trisomy 18 given this exact, connected combination.

D. This diagnosis carries a genuinely different, more limited prognosis than trisomy 21, requiring diagnosis-specific, honest counselling.

E. This family's own genuine values carry direct, essential relevance to this specific counselling conversation.

Board Alert Micrognathia, low-set ears, rocker-bottom feet, and clenched, overlapping fingers together are highly suggestive of trisomy 18, requiring honest, diagnosis-specific counselling regarding its more limited prognosis.

Question 24

A 24-week gestation infant is 6 weeks old and has developed significant, otherwise unexplained metabolic acidosis. On examination, this infant's abdomen is significantly distended with a faint, bluish discolouration of the abdominal wall. Which of the following best reflects the correct, connected diagnostic priority?

A. This finding carries no genuine, connected relationship to this infant's own underlying gastrointestinal status of any kind

B. This presentation should prompt urgent evaluation for necrotising enterocolitis with likely bowel ischaemia, since significant bowel ischaemia directly produces lactate accumulation through anaerobic metabolism, directly explaining this infant's own connected, significant metabolic acidosis together with this specific, concerning abdominal wall finding

C. This specific abdominal wall finding carries no genuine, diagnostic significance in this specific clinical context

D. This presentation should be managed exclusively as a primary respiratory disturbance, entirely unrelated to this infant's own abdominal findings

E. This infant requires no further, active or urgent evaluation of any kind

Answer: B. **This presentation should prompt urgent evaluation for necrotising enterocolitis with likely bowel ischaemia, since significant bowel ischaemia directly produces lactate accumulation through anaerobic metabolism, explaining this connected metabolic acidosis and abdominal wall finding.**

This vignette directly tests this book's own connected acid-base and surgical content: a bluish discolouration of the abdominal wall represents a genuinely concerning, specific physical examination finding directly suggesting significant, underlying bowel ischaemia or perforation, this same finding requiring urgent, active evaluation.

This same mechanism directly connects to this book's own foundational content regarding elevated anion gap metabolic acidosis: significant bowel ischaemia directly produces lactate accumulation through anaerobic cellular metabolism, as inadequate tissue oxygen delivery forces affected cells to shift away from normal, aerobic metabolism.

This reflects this book's own repeated theme that correctly, actively recognising significant, otherwise unexplained metabolic acidosis, together with a further, connected, concerning physical finding, should specifically, urgently prompt active consideration of this specific, genuinely serious gastrointestinal condition.

Why the other options are wrong

A. A direct, well-established, connected relationship exists between this finding and this infant's gastrointestinal status.

C. This specific finding carries direct, significant diagnostic significance in this specific clinical context.

D. This presentation is directly, connectedly related to this infant's own abdominal findings, not an unrelated respiratory disturbance.

E. This presentation warrants urgent, active evaluation, as detailed in the correct answer.

Board Alert A bluish abdominal wall discolouration with significant, otherwise unexplained metabolic acidosis should prompt urgent evaluation for necrotising enterocolitis with likely bowel ischaemia.

Question 25

A 27-week gestation infant is 5 weeks old and undergoing routine, structured iron deficiency screening using reticulocyte haemoglobin content, per a genuinely current quality improvement protocol. Screening reveals a low value. Which of the following best reflects the correct, connected clinical significance of this specific finding?

A. This finding carries relevance exclusively to this infant's own immediate haematological status alone, with no further, connected significance

B. This finding carries genuine, connected relevance to neuroprotection, since iron carries genuine, established importance for normal, healthy neurodevelopment, directly connecting this haematological finding to this infant's own broader, longer-term developmental outcome, supporting active, targeted treatment

C. This finding requires no further, active treatment or connected management of any kind

D. Iron carries no genuine, established relationship to neurodevelopment of any kind

E. This specific screening protocol carries no established basis in genuinely current literature of any kind

Answer: B. **This finding carries genuine, connected relevance to neuroprotection, since iron carries established importance for normal, healthy neurodevelopment, connecting this haematological finding to broader, longer-term developmental outcome and supporting active, targeted treatment.**

This vignette directly tests this book's own genuinely current care systems and quality improvement content: iron deficiency screening, established as part of a genuinely important, structured quality improvement initiative, carries direct, genuine, connected relevance to neuroprotection.

This same, specific mineral carries genuine, established importance for normal, healthy neurodevelopment, directly connecting this earlier case study's own specific, quality improvement target to a genuinely important, foundational physiological principle established elsewhere throughout this book, supporting active, targeted treatment once this specific deficiency is genuinely identified.

This reflects this book's own repeated theme that a specific quality improvement initiative's own genuine value frequently extends well beyond its own immediate, specific metric alone, to a further, genuinely important, connected physiological outcome directly relevant to this infant's own longer-term, connected trajectory.

Why the other options are wrong

A. This finding carries genuine, connected relevance extending beyond immediate haematological status alone, as detailed in the correct answer.

C. Active, targeted treatment is genuinely warranted once this deficiency is identified, as detailed in the correct answer.

D. A direct, established relationship exists between iron and neurodevelopment, as detailed in the correct answer.

E. This specific protocol has direct, genuine basis in genuinely current, published literature.

Board Alert Iron deficiency identified through structured screening carries genuine, connected relevance to neuroprotection, since iron carries established importance for normal, healthy neurodevelopment, supporting active, targeted treatment.

Question 26

A term infant born to a mother with confirmed, active genital herpes simplex virus infection, delivered vaginally, is currently asymptomatic at 24 hours of life. Which of the following best reflects the correct, current understanding of appropriate management in this specific circumstance?

- **A.** No specific, active management consideration is genuinely warranted, given this infant's own currently asymptomatic status
- **B.** Active, structured consideration of this infant's own elevated, connected transmission risk remains genuinely warranted, given this specific, high-risk delivery circumstance, supporting close, structured clinical monitoring for the subsequent development of significant, connected findings even in this infant's own current, asymptomatic state
- **C.** This infant's own currently asymptomatic status definitively excludes any further, genuine risk of subsequently developing this specific infection
- **D.** Maternal infection status carries no genuine relevance to correctly managing this specific, currently asymptomatic infant
- **E.** This specific delivery circumstance carries no genuine, connected relevance to this infant's own subsequent risk

Answer: B. **Active, structured consideration of this infant's elevated, connected transmission risk remains genuinely warranted given this high-risk delivery circumstance, supporting close, structured monitoring for subsequent development of significant findings even in this current, asymptomatic state.**

This vignette directly tests this book's own established infectious disease content regarding neonatal herpes simplex virus risk stratification: confirmed, active maternal genital infection at the time of vaginal delivery represents a specific, well-established, elevated transmission risk scenario, even in a currently, genuinely asymptomatic infant.

This means active, structured consideration of this infant's own elevated, connected risk remains genuinely warranted, supporting close, structured clinical monitoring for the subsequent development of significant, connected findings, since this infection can genuinely present later, beyond this infant's own initial, currently asymptomatic presentation.

This reflects this book's own repeated theme that correctly, safely managing a genuinely high-risk exposure requires active, structured, ongoing clinical vigilance, rather than assuming a currently asymptomatic presentation definitively, entirely excludes further, genuine risk.

Why the other options are wrong

A. Active, structured consideration remains genuinely warranted, given this high-risk circumstance, as detailed in the correct answer.

C. This current status does not definitively exclude further, genuine risk of subsequently developing this specific infection.

D. Maternal infection status carries direct, essential relevance to correctly managing this infant, as detailed in the correct answer.

E. This specific delivery circumstance carries direct, established relevance to this infant's own subsequent risk.

Board Alert Confirmed, active maternal genital herpes simplex virus infection at vaginal delivery warrants active, structured monitoring even in a currently asymptomatic infant, given genuine, elevated transmission risk.

Question 27

A 25-week gestation infant is 3 weeks old and has a significantly declining head circumference trajectory over the past 10 days, crossing two major percentile lines. Cranial ultrasound reveals evolving ventriculomegaly. Which of the following best reflects the correct, active, connected response to this specific combination of findings?

A. This combination of findings carries no genuine, connected significance, requiring no further, active evaluation

B. This combination warrants active, prompt, structured evaluation and close, ongoing monitoring, since these connected findings can reflect significant, underlying pathology requiring active, structured, longer-term neurodevelopmental follow-up regardless of this infant's own current, immediate clinical stability

C. Head circumference measurement carries no genuine, established relevance to this infant's own underlying neurological status

D. This infant's own current, stable, immediate clinical appearance definitively excludes the need for any further, active evaluation

E. Ventriculomegaly carries no genuine, connected relationship to this infant's own declining head circumference trajectory

Answer: B. This combination warrants active, prompt, structured evaluation and close monitoring, since these connected findings can reflect significant, underlying pathology requiring structured, longer-term follow-up regardless of current clinical stability.

This vignette directly tests this book's own established neurology content: a significant, declining head circumference trajectory, together with evolving ventriculomegaly on cranial ultrasound, together represent genuinely important, connected findings warranting active, prompt, structured evaluation.

This same, connected combination directly supports this book's own established, structured, longer-term neurodevelopmental follow-up programme, extending clinical attention well beyond this infant's own current, immediate clinical stability alone, given this specific pattern's own genuine, connected relevance to this infant's own longer-term developmental trajectory.

This reflects this book's own repeated theme that a specific, quantifiable clinical trend, correctly and actively monitored together with connected imaging findings, frequently provides genuinely important, connected diagnostic and prognostic information, regardless of whether this infant currently, immediately appears clinically well.

Why the other options are wrong

A. This combination carries genuine, connected significance, warranting active evaluation, not an absence of relevance.

C. A direct, established relevance exists between this measurement and neurological status, as detailed in the correct answer.

D. Current clinical stability does not exclude the need for further, active evaluation of this connected finding.

E. A direct, connected relationship exists between these two findings, as detailed in the correct answer.

Board Alert A significantly declining head circumference trajectory with evolving ventriculomegaly warrants active, structured evaluation and longer-term follow-up, regardless of current clinical stability.

Question 28

A 25-week gestation infant with confirmed, severe congenital diaphragmatic hernia and secondary persistent pulmonary hypertension, genuinely failing maximal conventional therapy, is being evaluated for ECMO. This infant is also extremely preterm with genuinely low birthweight. Which of the following best reflects the correct, connected synthesis of this circumstance's own competing considerations?

A. This infant's own extreme prematurity and confirmed, severe condition carry no genuine, connected relationship to one another of any kind

B. This infant's own confirmed, severe congenital diaphragmatic hernia with secondary persistent pulmonary hypertension represents a genuinely important, connected indication for ECMO, while this same infant's own extreme prematurity and genuinely low birthweight simultaneously represent a specific, relative contraindication given compounded bleeding vulnerability, requiring active, careful, individualised risk-benefit weighing rather than a single, automatic determination in either direction

C. This infant's own extreme prematurity should genuinely, automatically exclude any further consideration of this specific technology

D. This infant's own confirmed, severe condition should genuinely, automatically override any consideration of this infant's own extreme prematurity

E. This specific circumstance requires no genuine, active, individualised clinical judgment of any kind

Answer: B. **Confirmed, severe CDH with secondary pulmonary hypertension represents a genuinely important, connected ECMO indication, while extreme prematurity and low birthweight simultaneously represent a relative contraindication given compounded bleeding vulnerability, requiring careful, individualised risk-benefit weighing.**

This vignette directly tests this book's own established ECMO content, requiring genuine synthesis of two, genuinely opposing considerations together: confirmed, severe congenital diaphragmatic hernia with secondary persistent pulmonary hypertension, genuinely failing maximal therapy, represents a genuinely important, connected indication for this technology.

Simultaneously, this same infant's own extreme prematurity and genuinely low birthweight represent a specific, important relative contraindication, since this same technology's own genuine, required anticoagulation directly, considerably compounds this population's own already elevated, established bleeding vulnerability.

This reflects this book's own repeated theme that correctly, safely determining candidacy in this exact, genuinely challenging circumstance requires active, careful, individualised weighing of this connected risk against this technology's own genuine, potential benefit, rather than either consideration automatically, unilaterally determining this infant's own final candidacy alone.

Why the other options are wrong

A. A direct, connected, competing relationship exists between these two considerations, as detailed in the correct answer.

C. This prematurity represents a relative, not automatic, exclusionary contraindication requiring careful weighing.

D. This condition represents an important indication, not an automatic override of this infant's own connected, contraindicating risk.

E. Active, individualised clinical judgment is genuinely required in this specific, connected circumstance.

Board Alert Confirmed, severe CDH with secondary pulmonary hypertension is a genuinely important ECMO indication, while extreme prematurity and low birthweight simultaneously represent a relative contraindication — requiring careful, individualised weighing.

Question 29

A genuinely current, specific case-control study examines a rare, specific neonatal outcome, comparing affected cases against unaffected controls to identify a possible, connected exposure. Which of the following best reflects the correct, complete understanding of why this specific study design was likely chosen for this specific research question?

A. A cohort study would have provided an identical, equally efficient approach to studying this specific, rare outcome

B. A case-control study, in which individuals genuinely already carrying this outcome are genuinely compared against individuals genuinely without this outcome, frequently proves more efficient for studying a genuinely rare, specific outcome, since this same design genuinely avoids following a genuinely large, prospective cohort merely to observe a genuinely small number of this same, rare outcome eventually occurring

C. This specific study design carries no genuine, meaningful relationship to this specific outcome's own rarity

D. This specific study design choice carries no genuine, established rationale of any kind

E. A case-control study genuinely, characteristically follows a defined group forward over time from exposure toward outcome

Answer: B. **A case-control study frequently proves more efficient for studying a genuinely rare, specific outcome, since this design avoids following a large, prospective cohort merely to observe a small number of this rare outcome eventually occurring.**

This vignette directly tests this book's own foundational biostatistics content: a case-control study, in which individuals genuinely already carrying a given outcome are genuinely compared against individuals genuinely without this same outcome, looks backward toward a given, prior exposure, this same, backward-looking design genuinely well-suited to studying a genuinely rare outcome.

This specific distinction directly explains why a case-control study frequently, genuinely proves more efficient for studying a genuinely rare, specific outcome, since this same design genuinely avoids following a genuinely large, prospective cohort merely to observe a genuinely small number of this same, rare outcome eventually, genuinely occurring.

This reflects this book's own repeated theme that correctly, precisely selecting the appropriate, specific study design directly depends on the particular research question genuinely being asked, this same, efficient design choice directly informed by this specific outcome's own genuine rarity.

Why the other options are wrong

A. A cohort study would genuinely require considerably more resources to study this same, rare outcome efficiently.

C. A direct, meaningful relationship exists between this design and this outcome's own rarity, as detailed in the correct answer.

D. A direct, established, efficient rationale exists for this specific design choice, as detailed in the correct answer.

E. This reverses the correct relationship; a cohort study, not a case-control study, genuinely follows a group forward over time.

Board Alert A case-control study frequently proves more efficient for studying a genuinely rare outcome, avoiding the need to follow a large, prospective cohort merely to observe a small number of rare events.

Question 30

A 24-week gestation, small-for-gestational-age infant is 3 weeks old and has developed evolving bronchopulmonary dysplasia. This infant is also actively undergoing structured iron deficiency screening and has a family recently informed of a confirmed grade III intraventricular haemorrhage. Which of the following best reflects the correct, coordinated approach to this infant's own overall, connected care at this stage?

A. Each specific finding should genuinely be managed by an entirely separate, unconnected clinical team, without any genuine, coordinated, shared approach

B. This infant's care requires active, coordinated attention to the bidirectional, multifactorial bronchopulmonary dysplasia risk framework; connected, structured iron deficiency screening given its genuine relevance to neuroprotection; and honest, structured, longer-term neurodevelopmental follow-up given this infant's confirmed haemorrhage, together with honest, shared decision-making communication with this family throughout

C. This infant's own multiple, connected findings carry no genuine relationship to one another, requiring entirely separate evaluation

D. This family's own genuine values carry no genuine relevance to this infant's own overall, connected care

E. This genuinely complex circumstance can be correctly, completely managed without any genuine, coordinated, multidisciplinary discussion

Answer: B. This infant's care requires coordinated attention to the bidirectional BPD risk framework, connected iron screening given its neuroprotective relevance, and honest, structured follow-up given the confirmed haemorrhage — together with honest,

shared communication throughout.

This vignette directly tests genuine, cross-chapter synthesis: this infant's evolving bronchopulmonary dysplasia directly reflects this book's own established, bidirectional and multifactorial risk framework, requiring careful, ongoing ventilator and acid-base management.

This same infant's ongoing iron deficiency screening carries genuine, connected relevance to neuroprotection, while this infant's confirmed grade III intraventricular haemorrhage carries genuine, established relevance to longer-term neurodevelopmental outcome, requiring the same structured, longer-term follow-up this book establishes as essential.

This family deserves the same honest, shared decision-making conversation, honestly incorporating all of this connected, genuine uncertainty, that this entire book has modelled throughout its complete span, reflecting this book's repeated theme that coordinated, connected expertise represents the appropriate approach to this genuinely complex, multi-system circumstance.

Why the other options are wrong

A. A genuine, coordinated, shared approach, not entirely separate, unconnected teams, represents the correct approach.

C. These findings are directly, mechanistically connected to one another, as detailed in the correct answer.

D. This family's own genuine values carry direct, essential relevance to this infant's own overall care.

E. This genuinely complex circumstance requires coordinated, multidisciplinary discussion, not an absence of this coordination.

Board Alert Coordinated care for a critically ill, extremely preterm infant requires synthesising bidirectional BPD risk, connected neuroprotective screening, and honest, structured follow-up for significant IVH, together with honest family communication.

Mock Exam 3 — Section B: Organ Systems | Universal Task 3: Diagnosis, Testing and Monitoring

Question 31

A term infant develops significant jaundice on day 3 of life. Maternal blood type is A-positive, and infant blood type is O-positive. Direct antiglobulin testing is negative. Total bilirubin is significantly elevated with a direct fraction under

10 per cent. Which of the following best reflects the correct, connected diagnostic consideration this specific combination should prompt?

A. This presentation is definitively explained by ABO incompatibility, despite this infant's blood type and negative testing

B. This presentation is not consistent with ABO incompatibility, given this infant's own O-positive blood type and negative direct antiglobulin test, prompting active consideration of other, connected causes of significant, indirect hyperbilirubinaemia, including glucose-6-phosphate dehydrogenase deficiency or other, connected hemolytic processes

C. This infant's own specific blood type combination carries no genuine relevance to correctly interpreting this presentation

D. A negative direct antiglobulin test carries no genuine, diagnostic significance in this specific clinical context

E. This presentation requires no further, active diagnostic evaluation of any kind

Answer: B. **This presentation is not consistent with ABO incompatibility, given this infant's O-positive blood type and negative direct antiglobulin test, prompting active consideration of other causes of significant, indirect hyperbilirubinaemia, including glucose-6-phosphate dehydrogenase deficiency.**

This vignette directly tests correctly distinguishing ABO incompatibility from other, connected causes of significant hyperbilirubinaemia: ABO incompatibility specifically requires a genuine, antigenic mismatch, classically an O-positive mother with an A- or B-positive infant, together with a positive direct antiglobulin test confirming antibody-mediated hemolysis.

This infant's own O-positive blood type, genuinely identical antigenic status to the A-positive mother in the relevant, reverse direction, together with this infant's own negative direct antiglobulin test, directly excludes this specific mechanism, requiring active, further consideration of other connected causes of significant, indirect hyperbilirubinaemia.

This reflects this book's own repeated theme that correctly, precisely applying a specific, connected diagnostic framework requires actively confirming, rather than simply assuming, that a given infant's own specific laboratory findings genuinely, actually fit this same, initially suspected diagnosis.

Why the other options are wrong

A. This infant's specific blood type and negative testing directly argue against, not confirm, this specific diagnosis.

C. This specific blood type combination carries direct, essential relevance to correctly interpreting this presentation.

D. This negative result carries direct, significant diagnostic significance in this specific clinical context.

E. This significant presentation warrants active, further diagnostic evaluation, as detailed in the correct answer.

Board Alert ABO incompatibility requires an antigenic mismatch (classically O-positive mother, A- or B-positive infant) with a positive direct antiglobulin test — an O-positive infant with negative testing argues against this diagnosis.

Question 32

A 28-week gestation infant is 4 weeks old and remains on full parenteral nutrition with minimal enteral intake, having developed necrotising enterocolitis requiring bowel resection 2 weeks prior. Total bilirubin is now significantly elevated with a direct fraction of 55 per cent. Which of the following represents the correct, connected priority in this infant's own ongoing management?

A. This finding carries no genuine, connected relationship to this infant's own nutritional support of any kind

B. This finding is most consistent with parenteral nutrition-associated cholestasis, directly connecting to this infant's own genuinely prolonged parenteral nutrition duration following bowel resection, supporting active, careful consideration of advancing enteral feeds where genuinely, clinically possible given this infant's own reduced bowel length

C. This finding requires no further, active evaluation or connected management of any kind

D. This infant's own recent bowel resection carries no genuine relevance to this specific finding

E. This finding should be managed exclusively with continued, unchanged parenteral nutrition, without any genuine reconsideration

Answer: B. This finding is most consistent with parenteral

nutrition-associated cholestasis, connecting to this infant's genuinely prolonged parenteral nutrition following bowel resection, supporting careful consideration of advancing enteral feeds given reduced bowel length.

This vignette directly tests this book's own established nutrition content, now connected to this book's own surgical content: a predominantly direct hyperbilirubinaemia occurring in the setting of prolonged parenteral nutrition is most consistent with parenteral nutrition-associated cholestasis, this same risk directly elevated by this infant's own genuinely prolonged, connected treatment course following surgical bowel resection.

This infant's own reduced bowel length following resection directly complicates correctly, safely advancing enteral feeds, meaning this same, active consideration requires careful, individualised clinical judgment balancing this infant's own genuine need to reduce parenteral nutrition duration against this same, reduced bowel's own genuine, connected absorptive capacity.

This reflects this book's own repeated theme that correctly, actively managing a specific, connected nutritional complication requires active, individualised reconsideration of this infant's own overall feeding strategy, directly integrating this infant's own specific, connected surgical history.

Why the other options are wrong

A. A direct, established relationship exists between this finding and nutritional support, as detailed in the correct answer.

C. Active evaluation and connected management are genuinely warranted for this specific finding.

D. This infant's own recent resection carries direct, connected relevance to this specific finding and its management.

E. Active reconsideration of feeding strategy, not continued, unchanged parenteral nutrition alone, represents the correct approach.

Board Alert Parenteral nutrition-associated cholestasis following bowel resection requires careful, individualised consideration of advancing enteral feeds, balanced against reduced bowel length and absorptive capacity.

Question 33

A term infant develops ambiguous genitalia noted at birth. On day 5 of life, this infant develops significant vomiting, lethargy, and is found to have significant hyponatraemia and hyperkalaemia. Which of the following best reflects the correct, urgent, connected management priority?

A. This presentation carries no genuine, urgent significance of any kind, and evaluation can reasonably be deferred

B. This presentation represents a likely salt-wasting crisis in the setting of congenital adrenal hyperplasia, requiring urgent, immediate evaluation and treatment, including intravenous fluid resuscitation and stress-dose corticosteroid administration, given this specific presentation's own genuine, life-threatening potential

C. This specific electrolyte pattern carries no genuine relationship to this infant's own ambiguous genitalia

D. This presentation should be managed exclusively as a primary renal disorder, unrelated to any specific endocrine consideration

E. This infant's own ambiguous genitalia represents an isolated, unrelated, cosmetic finding requiring no further evaluation

Answer: B. **This presentation represents a likely salt-wasting crisis in congenital adrenal hyperplasia, requiring urgent, immediate evaluation and treatment, including intravenous fluid resuscitation and stress-dose corticosteroid administration, given genuine, life-threatening potential.**

This vignette directly tests this book's own established endocrine content regarding a genuine medical emergency: ambiguous genitalia combined with a significant, salt-wasting electrolyte pattern, hyponatraemia and hyperkalaemia together, directly reflects congenital adrenal hyperplasia due to 21-hydroxylase deficiency, now presenting in genuine, active salt-wasting crisis.

This specific diagnosis carries genuine, life-threatening urgency, since untreated salt-wasting crisis can rapidly progress to significant hypovolaemic shock, meaning correctly, rapidly recognising this connected presentation and initiating urgent evaluation and treatment, including intravenous fluid resuscitation and stress-dose corticosteroid administration, carries direct, potentially life-saving importance.

This reflects this book's own repeated theme that correctly, rapidly recognising a genuinely important, connected clinical pattern established at one point in a given infant's own course directly informs urgent, appropriate management once this same pattern's own genuine, active crisis subsequently, connectedly develops.

Why the other options are wrong

A. This presentation carries genuine, life-threatening urgency, not warranting deferred evaluation.

C. A direct, well-established, mechanistic relationship exists between this pattern and this infant's presentation.

D. This presentation reflects a significant, connected endocrine disorder, not a primary, unrelated renal disorder.

E. This finding carries direct, connected, urgent diagnostic significance, as detailed in the correct answer.

Board Alert Ambiguous genitalia with subsequent hyponatraemia and hyperkalaemia represents a likely salt-wasting crisis in congenital adrenal hyperplasia, requiring urgent fluid resuscitation and stress-dose corticosteroids.

Question 34

A Level II neonatal intensive care unit is planning a quality improvement initiative to improve outbreak preparedness. The team is designing this initiative's own outcome and process measures. Which of the following combined measures would most directly reflect this book's own established distinction between these two measurement categories?

A. A single, combined measure alone, without any genuine, meaningful distinction between process and outcome

B. A process measure tracking hand hygiene compliance, reflecting whether a specific, intended action actually occurred, together with an outcome measure tracking actual, connected infection rates, reflecting the genuine, clinical result this same action was ultimately intended to produce, actively tracked together since a genuinely improved process measure does not automatically guarantee a correspondingly improved outcome

C. Process measures and outcome measures reflect an identical, single specific category with no meaningful distinction

D. This specific initiative requires no genuine, structured measurement of any kind

E. Outcome measures alone provide an entirely complete, sufficient basis for evaluating this specific initiative

Answer: B. A process measure tracking hand hygiene compliance, together with an outcome measure tracking actual infection rates, should be actively tracked together, since a genuinely improved process measure does not automatically guarantee a correspondingly improved outcome.

This vignette directly tests this book's own foundational quality improvement methodology content: a process measure, generally reflecting whether a specific, intended action actually occurred, such as hand hygiene compliance, is genuinely, specifically distinct from an outcome measure, reflecting the actual, genuine clinical result this same action was intended to produce, such as actual infection rates.

This means correctly, completely evaluating this specific initiative requires actively tracking both of these genuinely different specific categories together, since a genuinely improved process measure does not automatically, reliably guarantee a correspondingly improved outcome measure, this same, connected principle directly extending this book's own established hand hygiene content from Volume 2's infectious diseases chapter.

This reflects this book's own repeated theme that correctly, honestly evaluating a given quality improvement initiative requires structured, comprehensive measurement extending beyond a single, isolated metric alone.

Why the other options are wrong

A. These reflect genuinely different, complementary specific categories, as detailed in the correct answer, not a single, combined measure.

C. These reflect genuinely different, specific measurement categories, as detailed in the correct answer, not an identical category.

D. This specific initiative genuinely benefits from structured measurement, as detailed in the correct answer.

E. Both categories together, not outcome measures alone, provide the genuinely complete, sufficient basis for evaluation.

Board Alert A process measure (hand hygiene compliance) and an outcome measure (actual infection rates) should be tracked together, since a genuinely improved process measure does not automatically guarantee a corresponding outcome improvement.

Question 35

A family whose infant has genuinely, actively been diagnosed with a significant, life-limiting condition is meeting with the clinical team to discuss neonatal organ donation as one, specific option they have heard about from another family. Which of the following best reflects the correct, complete, and coordinated approach to this specific conversation?

A. This specific topic should genuinely, never be discussed with any family under any circumstance

B. This specific consideration requires the same, careful, honest, and transparent approach this book establishes throughout as its own foundational, central approach, meaning correctly, compassionately discussing this specific, genuinely sensitive option with this family requires the same, careful attention to this family's own genuine values this book has emphasised throughout its entire content

C. This specific consideration should be approached with a genuinely different, less careful communication standard than the rest of this book's own content

D. This family's own genuine interest in this specific option carries no genuine relevance to correctly, compassionately responding

E. This specific consideration carries no genuine, established relationship to shared decision-making of any kind

Answer: B. This specific consideration requires the same careful, honest, and transparent approach this book establishes throughout as its foundational approach, with the same careful attention to this family's own genuine values.

This vignette directly tests this book's own established ethics content: neonatal organ donation represents a specific, genuinely important ethical consideration directly extending the shared decision-making content established throughout this book, this specific consideration genuinely requiring the same, careful, honest, and transparent approach.

This means correctly, compassionately discussing this specific, genuinely sensitive option with this family requires the same, careful attention to this family's own genuine values this book has emphasised throughout its own entire span, rather than this specific topic being treated as somehow separate or exempt from this book's own foundational communication standard.

This reflects this book's own repeated theme that its own foundational, shared decision-making approach applies with equal, genuine care to every specific, sensitive topic this book addresses, rather than this same, foundational approach being reserved for only certain, specific circumstances.

Why the other options are wrong

A. This specific option can genuinely, appropriately be discussed with an interested family, not universally excluded.

C. This same, careful communication standard applies consistently, not a genuinely different, less careful standard.

D. This family's own genuine interest carries direct, essential relevance to this conversation, as detailed in the correct answer.

E. This specific consideration has direct, essential relevance to shared decision-making, as detailed in the correct answer.

Board Alert Neonatal organ donation, when raised by a family, requires the same careful, honest, transparent, shared decision-making approach this book establishes as foundational to every sensitive topic it addresses.

Question 36

A genuinely current, specific randomised controlled trial enrolling preterm infants reports a genuinely current, specific number needed to treat of 25 for preventing a serious outcome. A second, separate trial examining a different intervention for the same outcome reports a number needed to treat of 8. Which of the following best reflects the correct, complete interpretation of these two, connected findings?

A. These two specific findings carry an identical, equally powerful clinical effect, with no meaningful, connected distinction between them

B. A genuinely lower number needed to treat directly reflects a genuinely more powerful, clinically important treatment effect, meaning the second intervention, requiring fewer patients treated to prevent one additional adverse outcome, demonstrates a genuinely stronger, connected clinical benefit than the first

C. A genuinely higher number needed to treat directly reflects a genuinely more powerful, clinically important treatment effect

D. This specific measure carries no genuine, meaningful relevance to correctly comparing these two, connected interventions

E. These two specific findings cannot genuinely, meaningfully be compared using this specific measure

Answer: B. **A genuinely lower number needed to treat directly reflects a genuinely more powerful, clinically important treatment effect — the second intervention, requiring fewer patients treated per outcome prevented, demonstrates a genuinely stronger clinical benefit.**

This vignette directly tests this book's own foundational biostatistics content regarding number needed to treat: this specific measure reflects the genuine number of patients who would genuinely need to receive a given intervention to prevent one, additional, genuinely adverse outcome.

This means a genuinely lower number needed to treat directly reflects a genuinely more powerful, clinically important treatment effect, meaning the second intervention, requiring only 8 patients treated compared with 25 for the first, demonstrates a genuinely stronger, connected clinical benefit for this same, shared outcome.

This reflects this book's own repeated theme that correctly, practically interpreting a given intervention's own genuine clinical value requires translating abstract, relative statistical measures into this same, genuinely intuitive, practical clinical language directly enabling meaningful comparison between two, genuinely different, connected interventions.

Why the other options are wrong

A. These two findings reflect genuinely different, connected clinical effects, as detailed in the correct answer.

C. This reverses the correct relationship; a genuinely lower, not higher, number reflects a more powerful treatment effect.

D. This specific measure carries direct, genuine relevance to comparing these interventions, as detailed in the correct answer.

E. These two findings can genuinely, meaningfully be compared using this specific, shared measure.

Board Alert A genuinely lower number needed to treat reflects a genuinely more powerful treatment effect — directly enabling meaningful comparison between two different interventions for the same outcome.

Question 37

A 26-week gestation infant develops a significant, new-onset seizure on day 6 of life. This infant's mother has confirmed, poorly controlled phenylketonuria and did not maintain dietary control during this pregnancy. Which of the following best reflects the correct, connected consideration this specific maternal history should prompt?

A. This maternal history carries no genuine, connected relevance to correctly evaluating this infant's own seizure of any kind

B. This infant's own presentation should prompt active consideration of maternal phenylketonuria syndrome, in which significant, uncontrolled maternal hyperphenylalaninaemia during pregnancy can directly produce significant, connected fetal and neonatal effects, including structural anomalies and neurological complications

C. Maternal phenylketonuria carries no genuine, established relationship to fetal or neonatal outcome of any kind

D. This presentation should be managed exclusively as idiopathic seizure, without any further, active diagnostic evaluation

E. This infant's own specific presentation carries no genuine, connected relationship to any specific, underlying metabolic consideration

Answer: B. This presentation should prompt active consideration of maternal phenylketonuria syndrome, in which significant, uncontrolled maternal hyperphenylalaninaemia during pregnancy can directly produce significant, connected fetal and neonatal effects, including neurological complications.

This vignette directly tests active, connected consideration of maternal phenylketonuria syndrome, a specific, genuinely important teratogenic effect in which significant, uncontrolled maternal hyperphenylalaninaemia during pregnancy directly crosses the placenta and can produce significant, connected fetal and neonatal effects.

This same, connected mechanism can directly produce structural anomalies, including significant cardiac and central nervous system malformations, together with significant, connected neurological complications, this infant's own seizure directly warranting active, structured evaluation given this specific, connected maternal history.

This reflects this book's own repeated theme that correctly, comprehensively evaluating a genuinely concerning presentation requires actively considering connected, relevant maternal history, rather than assuming every case of significant, neonatal seizure reflects an identical, unconnected, idiopathic process.

Why the other options are wrong

A. This maternal history carries direct, genuine relevance to this evaluation, as detailed in the correct answer.

C. A direct, established relationship exists between this maternal condition and fetal or neonatal outcome, as detailed in the correct answer.

D. This presentation warrants active, specific diagnostic evaluation, given this connected maternal history.

E. A direct, connected relationship exists between this presentation and this specific, underlying consideration.

Board Alert Poorly controlled maternal phenylketonuria during pregnancy can directly produce significant, connected fetal and neonatal effects, including structural anomalies and neurological complications, given significant hyperphenylalaninaemia.

Question 38

A 27-week gestation infant is 4 weeks old and remains on continuous positive airway pressure. This infant is being evaluated for possible retinopathy of prematurity and also has ongoing, structured screening for iron deficiency. The family asks whether these two, separate screening programmes are genuinely connected. Which of the following best reflects the correct, honest, complete response to this specific family question?

A. These two, specific screening programmes are genuinely, entirely unconnected in every respect, sharing no genuine, common purpose

B. While these two, specific screening programmes target genuinely distinct organ systems, they each directly reflect this book's own repeated, structured surveillance principle, applied consistently across multiple, genuinely important, high-risk considerations this population faces, each supporting this infant's own longer-term, connected wellbeing

C. This specific family question deserves no genuine, substantive, honest response of any kind

D. Structured surveillance carries no genuine, shared, underlying principle connecting these two, specific programmes

E. This infant's own gestational age carries no genuine relevance to either of these two, specific screening programmes

Answer: B. **These two programmes target genuinely distinct organ systems, but each directly reflects this book's own repeated, structured surveillance principle, applied consistently across multiple high-risk considerations, each supporting this infant's own longer-term wellbeing.**

This vignette directly tests this book's own repeated, cross-chapter demonstration of a shared, underlying principle: while retinopathy of prematurity screening and iron deficiency screening target genuinely distinct organ systems, both directly reflect this book's own repeated theme regarding structured, active surveillance for this population's own genuinely elevated, connected risk.

This same, shared principle directly connects to this book's own broader, repeated demonstration that a specific, high-risk population's own longer-term, connected developmental trajectory requires the same, structured surveillance principle, regardless of which specific organ system or condition this population's own particular, elevated risk actually originates from.

This reflects this book's own repeated theme that correctly, honestly answering a family's own genuine, thoughtful question requires actively connecting apparently separate, distinct clinical considerations back to this book's own shared, underlying, structural principle, rather than treating each specific screening programme as entirely, independently isolated.

Why the other options are wrong

A. A shared, underlying principle connects these two programmes, as detailed in the correct answer, not entirely unconnected purposes.

C. This specific family question deserves a genuine, substantive, honest response, as detailed in the correct answer.

D. A genuine, shared, underlying principle exists connecting these two programmes, as detailed in the correct answer.

E. This infant's own gestational age carries direct, genuine relevance to both of these screening programmes.

Board Alert Retinopathy of prematurity screening and iron deficiency screening target distinct organ systems but share this book's repeated, structured surveillance principle for this population's genuinely elevated, connected risk.

Question 39

A term infant develops significant respiratory distress and cyanosis at birth. Examination reveals a scaphoid abdomen and absent breath sounds on the left. The clinical team correctly avoids face mask ventilation and proceeds to immediate intubation. Which of the following best reflects the correct, connected rationale for this specific management decision?

A. Face mask ventilation carries no genuine, connected relationship to this infant's own specific presentation of any kind

B. This infant's presentation is consistent with congenital diaphragmatic hernia, and face mask ventilation is specifically avoided given the genuine risk of further gastric and bowel distension worsening pulmonary compression, since this same infant's herniated abdominal contents already occupy considerable, otherwise available thoracic space

C. Face mask ventilation represents the correct, preferred initial approach in every specific presentation, including this one

D. This infant's own specific presentation carries no genuine relevance to correctly selecting an appropriate mode of respiratory support

E. Immediate intubation carries no genuine, established rationale in this specific clinical circumstance

Answer: B. This presentation is consistent with congenital diaphragmatic hernia, and face mask ventilation is specifically avoided given the genuine risk of further gastric and bowel distension worsening pulmonary compression in this already thoracically crowded infant.

This vignette directly tests this book's own resuscitation content regarding a specific, important exception: this infant's presentation, a scaphoid abdomen and absent breath sounds on the left, directly reflects congenital diaphragmatic hernia, in which abdominal contents have herniated into the thoracic cavity.

Face mask ventilation is specifically avoided in this exact presentation, since positive pressure delivered through a mask directly risks further inflating the stomach and bowel loops already occupying thoracic space, directly worsening pulmonary compression in this same, already crowded thoracic cavity.

This reflects this book's own repeated theme that correctly, rapidly recognising a specific, connected clinical pattern directly changes the appropriate, immediate management approach, with immediate intubation representing the correct, preferred initial approach in this specific, recognisable presentation.

Why the other options are wrong

A. A direct, mechanistic relationship exists between face mask ventilation and this infant's presentation, as detailed in the correct answer.

C. This reverses the correct relationship; face mask ventilation should specifically be avoided in this presentation, not preferred.

D. This presentation carries direct, specific relevance to selecting the correct, appropriate mode of respiratory support.

E. A direct, established rationale exists for this specific approach, as detailed in the correct answer.

Board Alert Congenital diaphragmatic hernia: avoid face mask ventilation given risk of worsening gastric and bowel distension; proceed to immediate intubation instead, given already-compromised thoracic space.

Mock Exam 3 — Section C: Application | Universal Task 4: Management, Treatment and Prevention

Question 40

A 26-week gestation infant with confirmed, severe persistent pulmonary hypertension is being considered for ECMO. The clinical team debates central versus peripheral cannulation. Which of the following best reflects the correct, connected rationale generally favouring peripheral cannulation as the more common, initial approach?

A. Central and peripheral cannulation carry an identical degree of surgical invasiveness, with no meaningful, connected distinction between them

B. Peripheral cannulation, in which cannulae are placed through more accessible neck or groin vessels, generally represents the more common, initial approach given its own genuinely reduced surgical invasiveness compared with central cannulation's own considerably greater, direct surgical exposure requirement within the chest itself

C. Central cannulation generally represents the more common, initial approach given reduced surgical invasiveness, reversing the correct relationship established in this specific context

D. This specific distinction carries no genuine, meaningful relevance to correctly, appropriately selecting a given infant's own specific cannulation approach

E. Surgical invasiveness carries no genuine, meaningful relationship to either of these two specific cannulation approaches

Answer: B. **Peripheral cannulation, using more accessible neck or groin vessels, generally represents the more common, initial approach given its genuinely reduced surgical invasiveness compared with central cannulation's considerably greater, direct chest exposure requirement.**

This vignette directly tests this book's own established ECMO cannulation content: central cannulation, in which cannulae are genuinely, directly placed within the chest itself, generally through the great vessels adjacent to the heart, is genuinely, specifically distinct from peripheral cannulation, using more accessible neck or groin vessels.

Peripheral cannulation generally represents the more common, initial approach given its own genuinely reduced surgical invasiveness compared with central cannulation's own considerably greater, direct surgical exposure requirement, this same distinction directly relevant to correctly, safely planning this infant's own specific approach.

This reflects this book's own repeated theme that correctly, precisely characterising a given technical approach's own specific anatomical location directly informs the appropriate, individually tailored technique required, and why peripheral access is generally preferred as the initial, less invasive approach.

Why the other options are wrong

A. These two approaches carry a genuinely different, not identical, degree of surgical invasiveness, as detailed in the correct answer.

C. This reverses the correct relationship; peripheral, not central, cannulation generally represents the more common, initial approach.

D. This specific distinction carries direct, genuine relevance to appropriate approach selection, as detailed in the correct answer.

E. A direct, meaningful relationship exists between invasiveness and these approaches, as detailed in the correct answer.

Board Alert Peripheral cannulation, using more accessible neck or groin vessels, generally represents the more common, initial ECMO approach given genuinely reduced surgical invasiveness compared with central cannulation.

Mock Exam 3 — Section B: Organ Systems | Universal Task 3: Diagnosis, Testing and Monitoring

Question 41

A term infant develops significant respiratory distress, and echocardiography confirms hypoplastic left heart syndrome. This infant is started on prostaglandin E1 infusion. Which of the following best explains the correct, connected physiologic rationale for this specific intervention?

A. This medication carries no genuine, connected relationship to this infant's own specific cardiac lesion of any kind

B. This medication directly maintains ductal patency, this same, patent ductus arteriosus serving as this infant's own essential, connected pathway for systemic blood flow given this infant's own severely underdeveloped left-sided cardiac structures, meaning ductal closure would directly, rapidly prove fatal in this specific circumstance

C. This medication directly promotes ductal closure, the correct, opposite goal to what this infant's specific condition genuinely requires

D. Ductal patency carries no genuine relevance to this infant's own specific, connected cardiac physiology

E. This infant's own specific condition requires no further, active medication or connected management of any kind

Answer: B. **Prostaglandin E1 directly maintains ductal patency, this patent ductus arteriosus serving as this infant's essential**

pathway for systemic blood flow given severely underdeveloped left-sided structures — ductal closure would rapidly prove fatal.

This vignette directly tests foundational, connected cardiac physiology: in hypoplastic left heart syndrome, the left ventricle, aorta, and connected structures are severely underdeveloped, meaning this infant's own entire systemic blood flow genuinely depends on right-to-left flow through a patent ductus arteriosus.

Prostaglandin E1 directly maintains this same, essential ductal patency, this specific intervention directly preventing the normal, physiological ductal closure that would otherwise, rapidly occur following birth and prove genuinely, catastrophically fatal in this specific, duct-dependent circulation.

This reflects this book's own repeated theme that correctly, precisely understanding a specific, structural cardiac lesion's own genuine, connected physiology directly explains why a given, targeted medication represents essential, rather than optional, immediate management in this specific, life-threatening circumstance.

Why the other options are wrong

A. A direct, essential, mechanistic relationship exists between this medication and this infant's specific lesion.

C. This reverses the correct relationship; this medication maintains, not closes, ductal patency in this specific circumstance.

D. A direct, essential relationship exists between ductal patency and this infant's physiology, as detailed in the correct answer.

E. Active, immediate, targeted medication management is genuinely, essentially required for this specific condition.

Board Alert In hypoplastic left heart syndrome, prostaglandin E1 maintains essential ductal patency for systemic blood flow, given severely underdeveloped left-sided cardiac structures — ductal closure would rapidly prove fatal.

Mock Exam 3 — Section B: Organ Systems | Universal Task 4: Management, Treatment and Prevention

Question 42

A 29-week gestation infant is 2 weeks old and has developed significant abdominal distension with feeding intolerance. A specific, current guideline recommendation regarding peritoneal drainage versus laparotomy for this infant's suspected condition is under discussion. Which of the following best reflects the correct, honest understanding of the current evidence supporting these two, specific surgical approaches?

- **A.** High-certainty evidence has already, definitively established that one, specific approach is universally superior in every specific circumstance
- **B.** Genuinely current guideline evidence honestly acknowledges (very) low certainty of evidence regarding this specific comparison, meaning this decision genuinely requires dynamic, individualised clinical assessment rather than a single, universally validated recommendation
- **C.** This specific comparison carries no genuine, established basis in any current, published guideline of any kind
- **D.** This infant's own specific clinical trajectory carries no genuine relevance to this specific surgical decision
- **E.** Peritoneal drainage and laparotomy carry an identical, interchangeable clinical role in every specific circumstance

Answer: B. **Genuinely current guideline evidence honestly acknowledges (very) low certainty regarding peritoneal drainage versus laparotomy, meaning this decision genuinely requires dynamic, individualised clinical assessment rather than a single, universal recommendation.**

This vignette directly tests this book's own established surgical content regarding this book's own genuinely current, 2025 guideline: this same guideline honestly, transparently acknowledges (very) low certainty of evidence for the great majority of its own specific recommendations, including this exact comparison between peritoneal drainage and laparotomy.

This means correctly, safely deciding between these two, specific surgical approaches genuinely requires dynamic, individualised clinical assessment, actively integrating this infant's own specific, connected clinical trajectory, rather than a single, reliable, universally validated recommendation currently existing.

This reflects this book's own repeated theme of honest evidence treatment: even a genuinely current, structured guideline can honestly acknowledge genuine, remaining uncertainty in its own specific recommendations, reinforcing this book's repeated commitment to honest, complete treatment of genuinely current evidence.

Why the other options are wrong

- **A.** Genuine, low certainty exists for this specific comparison, as detailed in the correct answer, not definitively established superiority.

C. This specific comparison has direct, established basis in current, published guideline literature.

D. This infant's own clinical trajectory carries direct, genuine relevance to this specific decision.

E. These two approaches carry genuinely distinct, not interchangeable, roles requiring individualised, connected clinical judgment.

Board Alert Genuinely current NEC surgical guidelines honestly acknowledge (very) low certainty of evidence regarding peritoneal drainage versus laparotomy, requiring dynamic, individualised clinical assessment.

Question 43

A term infant develops significant, progressive respiratory distress and is noted to have significant polyhydramnios documented antenatally. At birth, an orogastric tube cannot be passed beyond a specific, resistance point, and this tube is noted to coil within the upper chest on radiograph. Which of the following best reflects the most likely, connected diagnosis?

A. This combination of findings carries no genuine, connected relationship to any specific, recognised congenital anomaly

B. This presentation is highly consistent with oesophageal atresia, most commonly with a connected tracheo-oesophageal fistula, this specific combination of antenatal polyhydramnios and this characteristic, bedside coiling sign together directly reflecting this specific, connected anatomic anomaly

C. This presentation is more consistent with congenital diaphragmatic hernia, which does not characteristically demonstrate this specific bedside finding

D. Polyhydramnios carries no genuine, connected relevance to this infant's own specific presentation

E. This specific bedside finding carries no genuine, diagnostic significance in this specific clinical context

Answer: B. **This presentation is highly consistent with**

oesophageal atresia, most commonly with a connected tracheo-oesophageal fistula — the antenatal polyhydramnios and characteristic, bedside coiling sign together directly reflect this specific, connected anatomic anomaly.

This vignette presents the classic, connected combination for oesophageal atresia: antenatal polyhydramnios, reflecting impaired fetal swallowing of amniotic fluid given this infant's own structurally interrupted oesophagus, together with the characteristic, bedside NG-tube-coiling sign directly reflecting this same, structural interruption.

This specific combination most commonly occurs together with a connected tracheo-oesophageal fistula, this book's own established surgical content directly connecting this specific anatomic combination to this infant's own genuine, elevated risk of aspiration and connected respiratory compromise.

This reflects this book's own repeated theme that correctly, precisely recognising a specific, characteristic bedside sign, together with connected antenatal history, directly supports rapid, confident diagnosis of this specific, genuinely important structural anomaly.

Why the other options are wrong

A. A direct, well-established, connected relationship exists between this combination and this specific, recognised anomaly.

C. This specific bedside finding, the NG-tube-coiling sign, is characteristic of oesophageal atresia, not congenital diaphragmatic hernia.

D. A direct, connected relevance exists between polyhydramnios and this infant's presentation, as detailed in the correct answer.

E. This specific finding carries direct, diagnostic significance in this connected presentation.

Board Alert Antenatal polyhydramnios with an NG-tube-coiling sign on radiograph is highly consistent with oesophageal atresia, most commonly with a connected tracheo-oesophageal fistula.

Question 44

A 26-week gestation infant is being managed on mechanical ventilation. The clinical team is discussing the correct, evidence-based rationale for permissive hypercapnia in this specific population. Which of the following best reflects the correct, honest, complete understanding of this specific approach's own evidence base?

A. This approach carries an entirely, definitively established upper carbon dioxide safety limit with no genuine, remaining uncertainty

B. Genuinely current trial evidence supports a higher, pH-controlled permissive hypercapnia target range as associated with increased ventilator-free days, without significant differences in bronchopulmonary dysplasia or evidence of neurodevelopmental harm, though this book honestly acknowledges the genuinely current absence of a formally established upper carbon dioxide safety limit

C. This specific approach carries no genuine, established evidence base of any kind

D. Ventilator-free days carry no genuine relevance to correctly evaluating this specific approach's own genuine benefit

E. This specific approach should genuinely, universally be avoided in every specific circumstance, given genuine safety concern

> Answer: B. **Genuinely current trial evidence supports a higher, pH-controlled permissive hypercapnia target as associated with increased ventilator-free days without significant BPD difference or neurodevelopmental harm, though this book honestly acknowledges the absence of a formally established upper safety limit.**
>
> This vignette directly tests this book's own established, honest acid-base content: a genuinely current, pH-controlled permissive hypercapnia randomised trial found a higher target range associated with increased ventilator-free days during the 28 days following randomisation, without significant differences in bronchopulmonary dysplasia or evidence of neurodevelopmental harm on follow-up.
>
> This same, genuinely current, honest acknowledgement directly extends to this approach's own remaining uncertainty: no formally established upper carbon dioxide safety limit currently, genuinely exists, meaning correctly, safely applying this approach requires continued, careful, individualised monitoring rather than either uncritical reassurance or universal avoidance.
>
> This reflects this book's own repeated theme of honest evidence treatment: genuinely current, positive trial evidence can coexist honestly alongside genuine, remaining uncertainty regarding this same approach's own precise, safe boundaries.

Why the other options are wrong

A. Genuine, remaining uncertainty exists regarding this upper limit, as detailed in the correct answer, not definitive establishment.

C. A direct, genuinely current, established evidence base exists for this specific approach, as detailed in the correct answer.

D. This specific outcome carries direct, genuine relevance to evaluating this approach's own benefit.

E. This approach carries genuine, evidence-supported benefit within an appropriate range, not universal avoidance.

Board Alert Genuinely current trial evidence supports a higher, pH-controlled permissive hypercapnia target associated with increased ventilator-free days, though this book honestly acknowledges the absence of a formally established upper safety limit.

Mock Exam 3 — Section B: Organ Systems | Universal Task 3: Diagnosis, Testing and Monitoring

Question 45

A term infant develops significant respiratory distress and cyanosis. Chest radiograph shows a 'boot-shaped' cardiac silhouette with decreased pulmonary vascular markings. Echocardiography confirms tetralogy of Fallot. Which of the following best explains this infant's own genuine risk during a significant, acute hypercyanotic episode?

A. This infant's own specific cardiac lesion carries no genuine, connected relationship to episodic, acute cyanotic events of any kind

B. A significant, acute increase in right ventricular outflow tract obstruction directly increases right-to-left shunting across this infant's own connected ventricular septal defect, directly, further reducing pulmonary blood flow and worsening this same, acute, connected cyanosis

C. This infant's own specific cardiac lesion carries an identical physiology to a lesion producing pulmonary overcirculation

D. Right ventricular outflow tract obstruction carries no genuine relevance to this infant's own connected cyanotic risk

E. This infant requires no further, active or urgent evaluation during any specific, acute cyanotic episode

Answer: B. A significant, acute increase in right ventricular outflow tract obstruction directly increases right-to-left shunting across the connected ventricular septal defect, further reducing pulmonary blood flow and worsening this acute, connected cyanosis.

This vignette directly tests foundational, connected cardiac physiology for tetralogy of Fallot: this specific lesion's own combination of right ventricular outflow tract obstruction, a ventricular septal defect, an overriding aorta, and right ventricular hypertrophy together create genuine, dynamic potential for episodic, acute worsening.

A significant, acute increase in this infant's own right ventricular outflow tract obstruction, whether through dynamic infundibular spasm or another, connected trigger, directly increases right-to-left shunting across this same, connected ventricular septal defect, directly, further reducing pulmonary blood flow and worsening this same, acute, connected cyanosis.

This reflects this book's own repeated theme that a specific, structural cardiac lesion's own genuine, connected physiology directly explains why this same lesion carries genuine, dynamic, and potentially acutely worsening risk, requiring active, urgent evaluation and management during any specific, significant hypercyanotic episode.

Why the other options are wrong

A. A direct, well-established, mechanistic relationship exists between this lesion and these episodic events.

C. This lesion carries a genuinely distinct physiology from pulmonary overcirculation, involving reduced, not increased, pulmonary flow.

D. A direct, mechanistic relationship exists between this obstruction and this infant's own cyanotic risk.

E. Active, urgent evaluation is genuinely warranted during any specific, significant hypercyanotic episode.

Board Alert In tetralogy of Fallot, a significant, acute increase in right ventricular outflow tract obstruction directly increases right-to-left shunting, further reducing pulmonary blood flow and worsening acute cyanosis.

Question 46

A 24-week gestation infant is being cared for at a Level III facility. The clinical team is discussing this infant's own overall care needs, including this book's own established, coordinated multidisciplinary care principle. Which of the following combined team members would most directly reflect this book's own comprehensive, coordinated approach to this infant's own care?

- **A.** A single, dedicated neonatologist acting entirely independently, without any further, coordinated, multidisciplinary involvement
- **B.** Neonatology addressing this infant's own broader, ongoing physiological status; nursing addressing continuous, structured bedside care; nutrition addressing this infant's own genuinely elevated, connected requirements; and structured, longer-term neurodevelopmental follow-up coordination, together reflecting this book's own repeated, coordinated care principle
- **C.** This infant's own care requires no genuine, coordinated, multidisciplinary involvement of any kind
- **D.** Nutrition carries no genuine, connected relevance to this infant's own overall, coordinated care team
- **E.** This infant's own care can be correctly, completely managed by any single, specific discipline acting entirely alone

Answer: B. **Neonatology, nursing, nutrition, and structured, longer-term follow-up coordination together reflect this book's own repeated, coordinated multidisciplinary care principle for this genuinely complex, extremely preterm infant.**

This vignette directly tests this book's own repeated, coordinated care principle, established throughout this entire book's own five-volume span: correctly, safely managing a genuinely complex, extremely preterm infant requires a coordinated, multidisciplinary team, rather than any single discipline acting entirely, independently alone.

This same, coordinated team directly spans neonatology addressing this infant's own broader, ongoing physiological status, nursing addressing continuous, structured bedside care, nutrition addressing this infant's own genuinely elevated, connected requirements established throughout this book's nutrition content, and structured, longer-term neurodevelopmental follow-up coordination.

This reflects this book's own repeated, closing theme that coordinated, connected expertise represents the appropriate approach to the genuinely complex clinical circumstances this book has demonstrated occur throughout the whole of perinatal and neonatal medicine, extending from this infant's own immediate, acute care through this same infant's own longer-term, connected trajectory.

Why the other options are wrong

A. This genuinely complex infant requires coordinated, multidisciplinary involvement, not a single discipline acting alone.

C. Genuine, coordinated, multidisciplinary involvement is genuinely required for this infant's own care.

D. Nutrition carries direct, essential relevance to this infant's own overall care team, as detailed in the correct answer.

E. This genuinely complex infant requires coordinated management, not management by a single discipline alone.

Board Alert Coordinated multidisciplinary care for an extremely preterm infant spans neonatology, nursing, nutrition, and structured, longer-term neurodevelopmental follow-up coordination together.

Mock Exam 3 — Section B: Organ Systems | Universal Task 3: Diagnosis, Testing and Monitoring

Question 47

A term infant develops significant vesicular skin lesions on day 5 of life. The mother reports no known history of genital herpes simplex virus infection, though this infant's presentation is genuinely concerning. Which of the following best reflects the correct, active diagnostic approach to this specific circumstance?

A. This infant's presentation should genuinely be dismissed, given this mother's own reported, negative history

B. Active, urgent evaluation for neonatal herpes simplex virus infection remains genuinely warranted despite this negative reported history, since a considerable proportion of maternal transmission occurs from mothers with genuinely unrecognised or asymptomatic infection, meaning a negative history does not entirely, reliably exclude this specific diagnosis

C. A negative maternal history definitively, completely excludes this specific diagnosis in every circumstance

D. This infant's own specific presentation carries no genuine, diagnostic significance given this reported, negative history

E. This presentation requires no further, active or urgent evaluation of any kind

Answer: B. **Active, urgent evaluation for neonatal herpes simplex virus infection remains genuinely warranted despite a negative reported history, since considerable transmission occurs from mothers with genuinely unrecognised or asymptomatic infection.**

This vignette directly tests an important, honest limitation of relying on maternal history alone: a considerable proportion of neonatal herpes simplex virus transmission genuinely occurs from mothers with genuinely unrecognised or asymptomatic infection at the time of delivery, meaning a negative reported history does not entirely, reliably exclude this specific diagnosis.

This infant's own genuinely concerning presentation, significant vesicular skin lesions, directly warrants active, urgent evaluation for this specific infection regardless of this negative reported maternal history, reflecting this book's own repeated theme that a given infant's own actual, presenting clinical findings frequently carry independent, genuine diagnostic weight.

This reflects this book's own repeated theme that correctly, comprehensively evaluating a genuinely concerning presentation requires active clinical judgment based on this infant's own actual findings, rather than relying exclusively on a potentially incomplete or unreliable maternal history alone.

Why the other options are wrong

A. This presentation warrants active, urgent evaluation despite this negative history, as detailed in the correct answer.

C. This negative history does not entirely, definitively exclude this specific diagnosis, as detailed in the correct answer.

D. This specific presentation carries direct, genuine diagnostic significance, regardless of this reported history.

E. This presentation warrants urgent, immediate evaluation, as detailed in the correct answer.

Board Alert A negative maternal history does not reliably exclude neonatal herpes simplex virus infection, since considerable transmission occurs from mothers with genuinely unrecognised or asymptomatic infection.

Question 48

A genuinely current survey has directly documented a significant nursing staff shortage across multiple neonatal intensive care units within a specific region. A specific Level III facility within this same region is considering whether to join a broader, coordinated network. Which of the following best reflects the correct, connected rationale supporting this specific decision?

A. This specific facility's own nursing shortage carries no genuine, connected relevance to this specific network decision

B. Neonatal intensive care unit networks represent a specific, genuinely important platform for continuous quality improvement, directly enabling systematic benchmarking and structured, mutual, collaborative learning across multiple, genuinely distinct facilities together, this same, coordinated structure potentially, directly supporting this specific facility's own connected, genuine staffing challenge

C. This specific facility should genuinely, always operate in complete isolation, without any genuine, coordinated network involvement

D. A coordinated, networked structure carries no genuine advantage over a single, isolated facility acting independently

E. This specific decision carries no genuine, established rationale of any kind

Answer: B. **Neonatal intensive care unit networks represent an important platform for continuous quality improvement, enabling systematic benchmarking and collaborative learning across facilities — potentially directly supporting this facility's own connected staffing challenge.**

This vignette directly tests this book's own established care systems content: neonatal intensive care unit networks, spanning genuinely broad regions, states, or entire countries together, represent a specific, genuinely important platform for continuous quality improvement.

This same, broad, connected structure directly enables systematic benchmarking, structured identification and implementation of best available evidence, and structured, mutual, collaborative learning across multiple, genuinely distinct facilities together, this same, coordinated approach potentially, directly supporting this specific facility's own connected, honestly acknowledged staffing challenge.

This reflects this book's own repeated, closing theme that safe, effective neonatal care depends not simply on individual clinical decision-making or even single-facility quality improvement alone, but on the broader, coordinated, networked systems within which this same care is actually, genuinely delivered.

Why the other options are wrong

A. This shortage carries direct, connected relevance to this network decision, as detailed in the correct answer.

C. A coordinated network, not complete isolation, represents the genuinely beneficial approach, as detailed in the correct answer.

D. A coordinated, networked structure provides genuine, established advantage, as detailed in the correct answer.

E. A direct, established rationale exists for this specific decision, as detailed in the correct answer.

Board Alert Neonatal intensive care unit networks represent an important platform for continuous quality improvement, potentially directly supporting a facility's own connected staffing challenges through coordinated, collaborative structure.

Question 49

A genuinely current, specific study reports its own primary result using a hazard ratio of 0.65 for a significant, time-to-event outcome. Which of the following best reflects the correct, complete interpretation of this specific measure?

A. A hazard ratio carries no genuine, meaningful relevance to correctly interpreting this specific finding of any kind

B. This hazard ratio of 0.65 reflects the genuine, relative rate at which this specific event genuinely occurs in the intervention group relative to the comparison group throughout a genuinely defined, continuous period of observation, this specific value directly suggesting a genuinely reduced rate of this event in the intervention group

C. This specific value carries no genuine relationship to this event's own specific timing of any kind

D. A hazard ratio and a relative risk reflect an identical, single specific measure with no meaningful distinction

E. This specific value directly suggests a genuinely increased, rather than reduced, rate of this event in the intervention group

Answer: B. This hazard ratio of 0.65 reflects the genuine, relative rate at which this event occurs in the intervention group relative to the comparison group over a defined period, directly suggesting a genuinely reduced event rate in the intervention group.

This vignette directly tests this book's own established biostatistics content regarding time-to-event research: a hazard ratio reflects the genuine, relative rate at which a given, specific event genuinely occurs in one, comparison group relative to another, throughout a genuinely defined, continuous period of observation.

This specific value of 0.65, being below 1.0, directly suggests a genuinely reduced rate of this event occurring in the intervention group relative to the comparison group, this specific measure genuinely, particularly useful when a given outcome's own genuine timing, not merely its own genuine, eventual occurrence, carries genuine, clinical importance.

This reflects this book's own repeated theme that correctly, completely understanding a given research finding requires actively selecting among this book's own multiple, genuinely distinct statistical measures, each carrying its own, genuinely different, appropriate interpretation and application.

Why the other options are wrong

A. This specific measure carries direct, genuine relevance to interpreting this finding, as detailed in the correct answer.

C. A direct, genuine relationship exists between this measure and this event's own specific timing.

D. These reflect genuinely distinct, connected specific measures, not an identical measure, as established throughout this book.

E. This value below 1.0 directly suggests a genuinely reduced, not increased, rate of this event.

Board Alert A hazard ratio reflects the genuine, relative rate at which an event occurs between groups over a defined period; a value below 1.0 directly suggests a genuinely reduced rate in the intervention group.

Question 50

A 25-week gestation infant has completed a 7-day continuous morphine infusion following significant abdominal surgery. The clinical team is planning discontinuation together with ongoing, structured pain assessment. Which of the following best reflects the correct, complete, connected approach to this specific transition?

A. This infusion should genuinely be discontinued abruptly, without any genuine, gradual, structured weaning process

B. This infant's own genuinely prolonged, 7-day infusion carries a genuine, significant risk of narcotic withdrawal symptoms upon discontinuation, requiring a genuinely gradual, structured weaning process together with continued, active pain and withdrawal assessment throughout this same, connected transition

C. This infant requires no further, active pain or withdrawal assessment once this infusion has been fully discontinued

D. Infusion duration carries no genuine, meaningful relationship to withdrawal risk in this specific circumstance

E. This specific consideration has no relationship to any established, current clinical guidance

Answer: B. **This infant's genuinely prolonged, 7-day infusion carries a significant risk of narcotic withdrawal symptoms upon discontinuation, requiring a gradual, structured weaning process together with continued, active pain and withdrawal assessment throughout.**

This vignette directly tests this book's own established pharmacology content: neonates genuinely treated with a continuous opioid infusion for a genuinely prolonged duration, established as approximately 5 days or considerably longer, are genuinely, significantly more likely to develop specific narcotic withdrawal symptoms once this infusion is genuinely, eventually discontinued.

This infant's own 7-day infusion duration directly exceeds this specific, practical threshold, meaning correctly, safely managing this specific circumstance requires actively, proactively anticipating this specific, connected withdrawal risk through a genuinely gradual, structured weaning process rather than abrupt discontinuation.

This reflects this book's own repeated theme that a specific medication's own genuine, connected risk frequently extends well beyond its own initial administration, requiring active, ongoing clinical attention throughout the entire, genuine duration of treatment and into its own eventual, careful discontinuation, together with continued, structured pain and withdrawal assessment throughout this same, connected transition.

Why the other options are wrong

A. Genuine, significant withdrawal risk exists, requiring a gradual, structured approach, not abrupt discontinuation.

C. Active, ongoing pain and withdrawal assessment remains genuinely important even following discontinuation.

D. A direct, established relationship exists between infusion duration and withdrawal risk, as detailed in the correct answer.

E. This specific consideration has direct, established basis in current clinical guidance, as detailed in the correct answer.

Board Alert A genuinely prolonged (approximately 5 days or longer) continuous opioid infusion requires a gradual, structured weaning process together with continued, active pain and withdrawal assessment throughout discontinuation.

Question 51

A family whose infant has genuinely, actively been redirected toward comfort-focused care is offered the option of postdeath cooling as part of comprehensive, compassionate bereavement care planning. Which of the following best reflects the correct, honest understanding of this specific consideration?

A. This specific consideration has no established basis in current, thoughtful literature addressing this field of any kind

B. Postdeath cooling represents a specific, genuinely important, practical consideration directly relevant to correctly, compassionately supporting a family's own genuine memory-making opportunities, this specific consideration representing a genuinely current ethical consideration directly identified within current, thoughtful literature addressing this field

C. This specific consideration carries no genuine relevance to correctly, compassionately supporting this family

D. Comprehensive, compassionate bereavement care requires no genuine, active familiarity with this specific, practical consideration

E. This specific consideration should genuinely, never be discussed with any family under any specific circumstance

Answer: B. Postdeath cooling represents a genuinely important, practical consideration directly relevant to supporting a family's own genuine memory-making opportunities — a genuinely current ethical consideration identified within thoughtful literature addressing this field.

This vignette directly tests this book's own established ethics content regarding a specific, practical consideration: postdeath cooling represents a specific, genuinely important, practical consideration directly relevant to correctly, compassionately supporting a family's own genuine memory-making opportunities.

This same consideration represents a specific, genuinely current ethical consideration directly identified within current, thoughtful literature addressing this field's own particular, practical complexity, meaning correctly, compassionately supporting a family requires active, informed familiarity with this specific, practical consideration.

This reflects this book's own repeated theme that comprehensive, compassionate bereavement care requires attention to specific, practical, and sometimes unfamiliar detail, alongside its own broader, emotional and ethical content, as one further, genuine dimension of comprehensive support.

Why the other options are wrong

A. This specific consideration has direct, genuine basis in current, thoughtful literature, as detailed in the correct answer.

C. This specific consideration carries direct, genuine relevance to compassionately supporting this family.

D. Active, informed familiarity with this consideration is genuinely important, as detailed in the correct answer.

E. This specific consideration can genuinely, appropriately be discussed as part of comprehensive bereavement care planning.

Board Alert Postdeath cooling represents a genuinely important, practical consideration supporting a family's own memory-making opportunities, identified within current, thoughtful literature addressing comprehensive bereavement care.

Question 52

A 30-week gestation infant develops significant, progressive abdominal distension on day 4 of life, notably earlier than typical necrotising enterocolitis presentation. This infant has not yet received significant enteral feeding and recently completed a course of postnatal dexamethasone together with indomethacin for a haemodynamically significant patent ductus arteriosus. Which of the following best reflects the most likely, connected diagnosis?

A. This presentation is most consistent with classic necrotising enterocolitis, sharing an identical mechanism, timing, and risk factor profile to this infant's own specific presentation

B. This presentation is more consistent with spontaneous intestinal perforation, a condition genuinely distinct from classic necrotising enterocolitis, given this infant's own connected, specific risk factors, including early postnatal corticosteroid exposure and concurrent indomethacin administration, together with this infant's own minimal enteral feeding history

C. This infant's own specific, connected risk factors carry no genuine relationship to this specific presentation

D. This presentation carries no genuine, connected relationship to this infant's own recent medication history

E. Enteral feeding status carries no genuine relevance to distinguishing between these two, genuinely distinct conditions

Answer: B. **This presentation is more consistent with spontaneous intestinal perforation, genuinely distinct from classic necrotising enterocolitis, given this infant's connected risk factors — early corticosteroid exposure and concurrent indomethacin — together with minimal enteral feeding history.**

This vignette directly tests correctly distinguishing spontaneous intestinal perforation from classic necrotising enterocolitis: this specific, distinct condition typically occurs earlier, often in infants not yet significantly enterally fed, carrying a genuinely different, specific underlying mechanism and connected risk factor profile.

This infant's own specific, connected risk factors, early postnatal corticosteroid exposure and concurrent indomethacin administration, have each been specifically associated with this distinct condition, directly connecting to this book's own established pharmacology content regarding indomethacin's own genuine, established connected risks.

This reflects this book's own repeated theme that correctly, precisely distinguishing between two, genuinely similar-appearing but mechanistically distinct conditions directly informs both correct diagnosis and appropriate, targeted management, given this infant's own specific, connected clinical and medication history.

Why the other options are wrong

A. This presentation's own timing and risk factors are more consistent with spontaneous intestinal perforation, a genuinely distinct condition.

C. These specific risk factors carry direct, established relevance to this presentation, as detailed in the correct answer.

D. A direct, established relationship exists between this presentation and this infant's own recent medication history.

E. Enteral feeding status carries direct, distinguishing relevance between these two, genuinely distinct conditions.

Board Alert Spontaneous intestinal perforation, genuinely distinct from classic necrotising enterocolitis, is associated with early postnatal corticosteroids and concurrent indomethacin, typically occurring earlier in infants not yet significantly fed.

Question 53

A 28-week gestation infant is 6 weeks old and has genuinely current, structured longer-term follow-up planning underway. The family asks how this specific programme relates to the extensive follow-up this book has established for infants with confirmed hypoxic-ischaemic encephalopathy or those supported on ECMO. Which of the following best reflects the correct, honest, complete response?

A. This specific programme carries no genuine, connected relationship to follow-up established for these other, connected populations

B. This same, structured, longer-term follow-up principle directly reflects the same, shared surveillance principle this book has established repeatedly for other genuinely important, high-risk neonatal populations, regardless of which specific condition originates their own, particular elevated risk

C. Extreme prematurity carries no genuine, connected relationship to any broader, shared surveillance principle of any kind

D. This specific family question deserves no genuine, substantive, honest response of any kind

E. Each specific high-risk population requires an entirely separate, unconnected follow-up principle with no genuine, shared structural basis

Answer: B. **This structured, longer-term follow-up principle directly reflects the same, shared surveillance principle this book has established repeatedly for other high-risk populations, regardless of which specific condition originates their elevated risk.**

This vignette directly tests this book's own repeated, cross-chapter demonstration: correctly, actively coordinating this infant's own genuinely current, structured follow-up with the extensive neurodevelopmental follow-up content established throughout this book for other genuinely important neonatal populations directly reflects a shared, structural principle.

This same, structured principle applies regardless of which specific, acute condition or intervention this population's own particular, elevated risk actually originates from, reinforcing this book's repeated, closing theme that a genuinely important, structural clinical principle continues to carry direct, connected relevance across the whole of neonatal medicine.

This reflects this book's own repeated theme that a specific, high-risk population's own longer-term, connected developmental trajectory requires the same, structured surveillance principle, whether this population's own elevated risk originates from extreme prematurity, hypoxic-ischaemic encephalopathy, ECMO support, or another connected, high-risk circumstance.

Why the other options are wrong

A. A genuine, shared, connected relationship exists across these populations, as detailed in the correct answer.

C. Extreme prematurity carries a direct, genuine relationship to this shared, broader surveillance principle.

D. This family's question deserves a genuine, substantive, honest response, as detailed in the correct answer.

E. A genuine, shared structural basis exists across these populations, not an entirely separate, unconnected principle for each.

> **Board Alert** Structured, longer-term neurodevelopmental follow-up reflects the same, shared surveillance principle across multiple high-risk populations, regardless of which specific condition originates their elevated risk.

Question 54

A term infant develops significant respiratory distress at birth, and physical examination reveals low-set ears, retrognathia, and bilateral talipes together with significant, symmetric growth restriction dating from early pregnancy. Which of the following best reflects the correct, connected diagnostic approach this presentation should prompt?

A. This combination of findings requires no further, active or structured diagnostic evaluation of any kind

B. This combination of three or more minor and major anomalies together should prompt active, structured evaluation for an underlying genetic syndrome, directly reflecting this book's own established dysmorphology principle that multiple, connected anomalies together significantly increase the probability of a major, underlying, connected condition

C. Growth restriction carries no genuine, connected relevance to this infant's own broader, structural evaluation

D. This specific combination of findings carries no genuine, established relationship to any broader, connected genetic evaluation

E. This infant's own specific presentation should be evaluated as entirely, individually isolated findings, without any genuine, connected consideration

> **Answer: B. This combination of three or more minor and major anomalies together should prompt active, structured evaluation for an underlying genetic syndrome, reflecting this book's established dysmorphology principle that multiple, connected anomalies significantly increase major-condition probability.**
>
> This vignette directly tests this book's own established, foundational dysmorphology principle: three or more minor anomalies together significantly increase the probability of an underlying, connected major anomaly or genetic syndrome, this same principle directly applicable to this infant's own connected combination of findings.

This infant's own combination of low-set ears, retrognathia, bilateral talipes, and early, symmetric growth restriction together directly warrants active, structured genetic evaluation, rather than each specific finding being considered an entirely isolated, unconnected observation.

This reflects this book's own repeated theme that correctly, comprehensively evaluating a genuinely concerning presentation requires actively recognising connected, multiple findings as a genuine, structured pattern, directly informing appropriate, comprehensive diagnostic evaluation extending well beyond any single, presenting finding alone.

Why the other options are wrong

A. This combination warrants active, structured diagnostic evaluation, not an absence of further consideration.

C. Growth restriction carries direct, connected relevance to this infant's own broader evaluation, as detailed in the correct answer.

D. A direct, established relationship exists between this combination and broader genetic evaluation, as detailed in the correct answer.

E. These findings should genuinely be evaluated together as a connected pattern, not entirely, individually isolated.

Board Alert Three or more minor and major anomalies together significantly increase the probability of an underlying, connected genetic syndrome, warranting active, structured diagnostic evaluation rather than isolated consideration.

Question 55

A 25-week gestation infant with confirmed, severe persistent pulmonary hypertension is being considered for ECMO. The clinical team calculates a specific oxygenation index and separately considers this infant's own extreme prematurity as a relative contraindication. The family asks how these two, separate considerations relate to one another. Which of the following best reflects the correct, complete, and honest response to this specific question?

A. These two considerations carry no genuine, connected relationship to one another of any kind

B. The oxygenation index provides a specific, quantified measure of this infant's own respiratory failure severity directly informing candidacy, while this infant's own extreme prematurity separately represents a relative contraindication given compounded bleeding vulnerability, meaning correctly, safely determining this infant's own overall candidacy requires actively, together weighing both of these genuinely distinct, connected considerations

C. The oxygenation index alone provides an entirely complete, sufficient basis for this infant's own candidacy determination

D. This infant's own extreme prematurity carries no genuine relevance to this infant's own overall candidacy determination

E. This specific family question deserves no genuine, substantive, honest response of any kind

Answer: B. The oxygenation index provides a quantified measure of respiratory failure severity informing candidacy, while extreme prematurity separately represents a relative contraindication given compounded bleeding vulnerability — both genuinely distinct considerations must be weighed together.

This vignette directly tests genuine synthesis of this book's own established ECMO fundamentals content: the oxygenation index, directly incorporating mean airway pressure, fraction of inspired oxygen, and arterial oxygen tension together, provides a specific, quantified measure of the genuine severity of this infant's own respiratory failure, directly informing candidacy.

This infant's own extreme prematurity separately represents a specific, important relative contraindication, since this same technology's own genuine, required anticoagulation directly, considerably compounds this population's own already elevated, established bleeding vulnerability, this specific consideration genuinely distinct from, though connected to, this infant's own quantified respiratory severity.

This means correctly, safely determining this infant's own overall candidacy requires actively, together weighing both of these genuinely distinct, connected considerations, reinforcing this book's repeated theme that correctly, safely applying this technology requires structured, quantitative assessment together with active, individualised risk-benefit weighing, rather than either consideration evaluated in complete isolation.

Why the other options are wrong

A. A genuine, connected relationship exists between these two considerations, as detailed in the correct answer.

C. This index alone does not provide a complete basis; extreme prematurity must also be actively considered together.

D. This infant's own extreme prematurity carries direct, genuine relevance to this overall determination.

E. This specific family question deserves a genuine, substantive, honest response, as detailed in the correct answer.

Board Alert ECMO candidacy requires together weighing the quantified oxygenation index (respiratory severity) and extreme prematurity's own relative contraindication (compounded bleeding vulnerability) as genuinely distinct, connected considerations.

Question 56

A term infant develops significant respiratory distress at birth and is found to have a large, left-sided pneumothorax on chest radiograph, together with a history of significant, prolonged rupture of membranes and clinical signs concerning for significant chorioamnionitis. Which of the following best reflects the correct, connected approach to this infant's own overall management?

A. This infant's pneumothorax and this infant's own connected infectious risk should be managed as entirely separate, unconnected clinical problems

B. This infant requires both active, immediate decompression of this significant pneumothorax and active, prompt evaluation for early-onset sepsis, including blood culture and empiric antibiotic therapy, given this infant's own connected, elevated infectious risk profile, these two, genuinely important considerations requiring simultaneous, coordinated attention

C. This infant's own connected infectious risk carries no genuine relevance to this infant's own respiratory management

D. This infant's own significant pneumothorax carries no genuine, urgent significance in this specific clinical context

E. This infant requires no further, active or urgent evaluation of any kind, given this infant's own current presentation

Answer: B. This infant requires both active, immediate pneumothorax decompression and prompt evaluation for early-onset sepsis, given this connected, elevated infectious risk profile — these two important considerations require simultaneous, coordinated attention.

This vignette directly tests genuine, simultaneous synthesis of two, connected clinical priorities this book has established throughout: a significant, symptomatic pneumothorax requires active, immediate decompression, this same, genuinely urgent intervention not diminished by this infant's own additional, connected infectious risk.

This infant's own significant, connected history of prolonged rupture of membranes and clinical chorioamnionitis simultaneously represents a genuinely elevated, connected risk profile for early-onset sepsis, requiring active, prompt evaluation, including blood culture and empiric antibiotic therapy, alongside this infant's own respiratory management.

This reflects this book's own repeated theme that correctly, safely managing a genuinely complex, multi-system presentation requires active, simultaneous, coordinated attention to multiple, genuinely important, connected clinical priorities together, rather than addressing each specific finding sequentially, in complete isolation from the other.

Why the other options are wrong

A. These two considerations require simultaneous, coordinated attention, not entirely separate, unconnected management.

C. This risk carries direct, connected relevance to this infant's own overall management, alongside respiratory care.

D. This pneumothorax carries genuine, urgent significance requiring active, immediate decompression.

E. This infant requires active, urgent evaluation across multiple, connected priorities, as detailed in the correct answer.

Board Alert A significant pneumothorax together with an elevated, connected sepsis risk profile requires simultaneous, coordinated attention — active, immediate decompression alongside prompt sepsis evaluation and empiric treatment.

Question 57

A genuinely current, specific quality improvement initiative reports a significant improvement in screening rates after excluding infants who genuinely died or were genuinely transferred before eligibility for the specific outcome being measured. Which of the following best reflects the correct, complete understanding of why this specific methodological step was genuinely necessary?

A. This specific methodological step carries no genuine relevance to correctly, accurately interpreting this initiative's own reported screening rate

B. Correctly, accurately interpreting this same, quality improvement initiative's own actual, genuine screening rate requires actively applying clearly defined, specific exclusion criteria, rather than including every specific infant admitted regardless of this same infant's own actual eligibility for the specific outcome genuinely being measured

C. Every specific infant admitted should genuinely be included in this same, calculated rate, regardless of this same infant's own actual eligibility

D. Death or genuine transfer before eligibility carries no genuine, meaningful relevance to correctly, accurately calculating this specific rate

E. This specific methodological step has no established basis in genuinely current, recognised quality improvement literature

Answer: B. **Correctly, accurately interpreting this initiative's own actual screening rate requires clearly defined, specific exclusion criteria, rather than including every admitted infant regardless of actual eligibility for the specific outcome being measured.**

This vignette directly tests this book's own established quality improvement methodology content: correctly, actively excluding an infant who genuinely dies or is genuinely transferred before eligibility represents a genuinely important, specific methodological consideration directly relevant to this initiative's own accurate, honest reporting.

This means correctly, accurately interpreting this same, quality improvement initiative's own actual, genuine screening rate requires actively applying clearly defined, specific exclusion criteria, rather than including every specific infant admitted regardless of this same infant's own actual eligibility for the specific outcome genuinely being measured.

This reflects this book's own repeated theme that correctly, honestly evaluating a given quality improvement initiative requires structured, precise methodology at every genuine stage, including this same initiative's own specific, defined population, rather than a potentially misleading, unadjusted rate.

Why the other options are wrong

A. This specific methodological step carries direct, essential relevance to correctly interpreting this rate, as detailed in the correct answer.

C. Clearly defined exclusion criteria, not universal inclusion, represent the correct, accurate methodological approach.

D. A direct, meaningful relevance exists between this and accurate rate calculation, as detailed in the correct answer.

E. This specific methodological step has direct, genuine basis in current, recognised quality improvement literature.

Board Alert Correctly, accurately interpreting a quality improvement initiative's screening rate requires clearly defined exclusion criteria for infants who died or were transferred before eligibility, not universal inclusion regardless of eligibility.

Question 58

A 24-week gestation infant is receiving structured, validated pain and sedation scoring throughout an extended hospitalisation. The family asks why this book emphasises structured scoring over clinical impression alone. Which of the following best reflects the correct, honest, complete response to this specific family question?

A. Clinical impression alone provides an entirely sufficient, equally reliable approach, making structured scoring genuinely unnecessary

B. A specific, validated pain and sedation scoring tool provides a genuinely important, structured, and considerably more objective approach to guiding sedation and analgesia decisions than clinical impression alone, this same, structured approach directly reducing genuine, subjective variability between different, individual clinicians assessing this same infant

C. This specific family question deserves no genuine, substantive, honest response of any kind

D. Structured scoring carries no genuine, meaningful advantage over clinical impression alone in any specific circumstance

E. This infant's own specific, individual circumstance carries no genuine relevance to this specific comparison

Answer: B. A validated pain and sedation scoring tool provides a genuinely more objective approach than clinical impression alone, directly reducing genuine, subjective variability between different, individual clinicians assessing the same infant.

This vignette directly tests this book's own established pharmacology content, now framed as an honest, direct family response: correctly, actively using a specific, validated pain and sedation scoring tool provides a genuinely important, structured, and considerably more objective approach to guiding sedation and analgesia decisions than clinical impression alone.

This same, structured approach directly reduces genuine, subjective variability that can genuinely occur between different, individual clinicians each independently assessing this same infant, this same, reduced variability directly supporting more consistent, reliable, and safer clinical decision-making across this infant's own entire, extended hospitalisation.

This reflects this book's own repeated theme that correctly, safely applying sedation and analgesia in this genuinely vulnerable population requires structured, objective clinical assessment, this same, honest rationale representing exactly the kind of clear, substantive response this book has modelled throughout for genuine, thoughtful family questions.

Why the other options are wrong

A. A specific, validated tool provides genuine, additional, objective value, as detailed in the correct answer, not equal sufficiency.

C. This specific family question deserves a genuine, substantive, honest response, as detailed in the correct answer.

D. A genuine, meaningful advantage exists for structured scoring, as detailed in the correct answer.

E. This infant's own specific circumstance carries direct, genuine relevance to this comparison, as detailed in the correct answer.

Board Alert A validated pain and sedation scoring tool provides a genuinely more objective approach than clinical impression alone, directly reducing subjective variability between different clinicians assessing the same infant.

Question 59

A genuinely current, specific systematic review pooling data from multiple studies of a perinatal intervention reports a pooled effect estimate with a genuinely narrow 95 per cent confidence interval, entirely excluding the null value. Which of the following best reflects the correct, complete, and honest interpretation of this specific finding?

A. This finding should genuinely, uncritically be accepted as entirely, definitively conclusive, with no further, critical consideration of any kind

B. This genuinely narrow confidence interval reflects genuinely greater precision in this pooled estimate, though correctly, completely evaluating this same finding still requires actively considering this same review's own genuine, potential publication bias and the genuine, underlying quality and consistency of the individual, pooled studies together

C. A genuinely narrow confidence interval carries an identical, equally imprecise meaning to a genuinely wide confidence interval

D. This specific interval's own reported width has no genuine relationship to this review's own genuine, underlying precision

E. This specific finding carries no genuine, remaining limitation of any kind, given this genuinely narrow interval

Answer: B. **This genuinely narrow confidence interval reflects greater precision, though complete evaluation still requires actively considering this review's own genuine, potential publication bias and the underlying quality and consistency of the pooled studies together.**

This vignette directly tests genuine synthesis of this book's own established biostatistics content across multiple subdomains: a genuinely narrow confidence interval directly reflects genuinely greater precision in this pooled estimate, this specific interpretation directly extending this book's own established confidence interval content.

This means correctly, completely evaluating this same finding still requires actively considering this same review's own genuine, potential publication bias, this book's own established limitation directly relevant to any systematic review or meta-analysis, together with the genuine, underlying quality and consistency of the individual, pooled studies.

This reflects this book's own repeated, closing theme that correctly, critically appraising even a genuinely precise, statistically significant pooled finding requires active, ongoing attention to this same finding's own genuine, connected methodological limitation, rather than uncritical, complete acceptance regardless of these important, connected considerations.

Why the other options are wrong

A. Genuine, remaining critical consideration is required, as detailed in the correct answer, not uncritical, definitive acceptance.

C. A genuinely narrow interval reflects genuinely different, more precise meaning compared with a genuinely wide interval.

D. A direct, genuine relationship exists between interval width and precision, as detailed in the correct answer.

E. Genuine, remaining limitation exists, as detailed in the correct answer, even with this genuinely narrow interval.

Board Alert A genuinely narrow confidence interval reflects greater precision, but complete evaluation of a pooled estimate still requires active consideration of publication bias and the underlying quality of pooled studies.

Question 60

This is the final question of Mock Exam 3, and the final question of this entire book's own five-volume, integrated question bank. A 24-week gestation infant with confirmed, severe congenital diaphragmatic hernia and secondary persistent pulmonary hypertension, genuinely failing maximal conventional therapy, is being evaluated for ECMO at a referring, Level II facility. This infant's family is present, asking detailed questions about this proposed intervention's genuine risk, while the clinical team simultaneously debates cannulation approach given genuinely current, portable technology, this infant's own extreme prematurity, and this infant's own eventual need for coordinated, structured, longer-term follow-up. Which of the following best reflects the complete, correct, and fully coordinated approach to this entire, connected circumstance?

A. Each specific consideration should genuinely be addressed by an entirely separate, unconnected team, without any genuine, coordinated, shared approach with this family

B. Recognise that this infant's own confirmed, severe condition represents a genuinely important, connected ECMO indication, while this infant's own extreme prematurity simultaneously represents a specific, relative contraindication requiring careful, individualised risk-benefit weighing; recognise that genuinely current, portable technology may enable safe, on-site cannulation before transport, requiring the specialised, coordinated mobile ECMO team this circumstance demands; recognise that correctly, safely applying this technology requires the coordinated, multidisciplinary team and active neuromonitoring this entire book establishes throughout; recognise that this infant's eventual, structured, longer-term follow-up reflects the same, shared surveillance principle this book has established repeatedly; and recognise that this family's detailed questions deserve the same honest, calibrated, shared decision-making communication this entire book has modelled throughout its complete, five-volume span

C. This infant's own extremely preterm status carries no genuine relevance to correctly determining candidacy for this technology

D. This family's own detailed questions should genuinely, entirely be deferred until this specific procedure has already, fully concluded

E. This genuinely complex, combined circumstance can be correctly, safely managed by a single specialist acting entirely independently, without genuine, coordinated involvement of any kind

Answer: B. **Every principle across this entire five-volume book converges here: the connected ECMO indication and relative contraindication requiring careful weighing, genuinely current transport technology, coordinated technical management and neuromonitoring, structured longer-term follow-up, and honest, shared family communication — the complete, connected standard this entire book has been built toward.**

This truly final question of this entire book's own integrated question bank is deliberately constructed to require synthesis across essentially every domain this book has addressed across its complete, five-volume span — foundational physiology, connected organ systems, surgical and technological application, ethics, and biostatistics together.

This infant's own confirmed, severe condition directly represents a genuinely important, connected ECMO indication, while this infant's own extreme prematurity simultaneously represents a specific, relative contraindication given compounded bleeding vulnerability, requiring careful, individualised risk-benefit weighing; genuinely current, portable technology may enable safe, on-site cannulation, requiring the specialised, coordinated mobile ECMO team this circumstance demands; and correctly, safely applying this technology requires the coordinated, multidisciplinary team and active neuromonitoring this entire book establishes throughout.

This infant's own eventual, structured, longer-term follow-up directly reflects the same, shared surveillance principle this book has established repeatedly across every genuinely important, high-risk population it has addressed, while this family's own detailed, difficult questions deserve the same honest, calibrated, shared decision-making communication this entire book has modelled throughout its complete, five-volume span — closing this entire book's own question bank on precisely the standard of connected, compassionate, and rigorous synthesis this entire project has been built toward from its very first question.

Why the other options are wrong

A. A genuine, coordinated, shared approach, not entirely separate, unconnected teams, represents the correct approach.

C. This specific status carries direct, particular relevance to determining candidacy, as detailed in the correct answer.

D. This family deserves honest, timely communication throughout this process, not deferral until after this procedure concludes.

E. This genuinely complex circumstance requires coordinated, multidisciplinary management, not a single specialist acting independently.

Board Alert This is the truly final question of this entire, five-volume question bank, deliberately constructed to require synthesis of every major theme this book has addressed across its complete span.

Score Tracker: Mock Examination 3

Record your score by section below, and compare across all three mock examinations for your final, complete picture.

A Closing Note

This is the final mock examination in this book. If you have worked through all three, you have now practised applying this book's own connected reasoning across 180 genuinely independent clinical vignettes, spanning every domain this book has addressed across its complete, five-volume span.

The reference ranges appendix that follows this exam is a quick-reference tool, not a teaching chapter — use it as a bedside companion during your remaining preparation, and during your actual clinical practice afterward.

Whatever the specific date of your own certifying examination, the method this book has taught throughout — mechanism first, honest about uncertainty, connected across chapters and volumes — will continue to serve you well beyond it.

Chapter: Suggested Reading and Valuable Resources

This book was built as a complete, standalone review resource, but no single book, however comprehensive, should be a candidate's only source across an entire preparation period. The resources below are widely used, established references in neonatal-perinatal medicine, offered here as a starting point for deeper reading on any topic where this book's own coverage leaves you wanting more — not as a required reading list, and not as an exhaustive one.

1. Core Reference Textbooks

Title	Best used for
Fanaroff and Martin's Neonatal-Perinatal Medicine: Diseases of the Fetus and Infant	The most comprehensive, widely cited single reference in the field; strongest as a deep-dive resource for a specific topic rather than cover-to-cover reading.
Avery's Diseases of the Newborn	A long-standing, authoritative core text with strong pathophysiological grounding, complementary to this book's own mechanism-first approach.
Cloherty and Stark's Manual of Neonatal Care	A genuinely practical, bedside-oriented manual; strong for translating principles into concrete, protocol-level management.
Gomella's Neonatology: Management, Procedures, On-Call Problems, Diseases, and Drugs	Particularly useful as a quick, structured reference during clinical rotations, organised around common on-call scenarios.
Rennie and Roberton's Textbook of Neonatology	A well-regarded, UK-originated core text with particular strength in physiology and evidence-based practice.

2. Journals Worth Following

Journal	Focus
Journal of Perinatology	Clinical and translational perinatal-neonatal research; a strong source for exactly the kind of genuinely current findings this book has drawn on throughout.
Pediatrics (American Academy of Pediatrics)	Broad paediatric research and policy, including regularly updated AAP clinical guidance directly relevant to neonatal practice.
NeoReviews	An AAP-published, education-focused journal specifically designed for trainees and board preparation; frequently the most directly relevant single journal for exam-style review.
Archives of Disease in Childhood – Fetal and Neonatal Edition	Strong, UK- and Europe-originated neonatal and perinatal research, complementing the more US-centred sources above.
Seminars in Perinatology	Themed issues offering deep, focused reviews of a single topic area — useful for building genuine depth once foundational knowledge is secure.
The Journal of Pediatrics	Broad paediatric clinical research with a substantial, regular neonatal component.

3. Guidelines and Professional Bodies

Organisation	Why it matters
American Academy of Pediatrics (AAP)	Publishes the great majority of US clinical practice guidelines directly relevant to neonatal care, updated on an ongoing basis — always worth checking for the most current version of a specific guideline.
American College of Obstetricians and Gynecologists (ACOG)	The primary source for maternal-fetal medicine guidance, directly relevant to this book's own Volume 1 content and every antenatal counselling scenario throughout.
Extracorporeal Life Support Organization (ELSO)	The primary, international source for ECMO-specific guidelines, registry data, and training standards — directly relevant to this book's own Volume 4 transport and ECMO chapter.
Neonatal Resuscitation Program (NRP)	The AAP- and American Heart Association-affiliated source for the current resuscitation algorithm this book has referenced throughout its own delivery room content.
Cochrane Neonatal	A specific, focused branch of the Cochrane systematic review collaboration; an excellent source for genuinely current, rigorously appraised evidence on a specific, narrow clinical question.

4. Point-of-Care and Ongoing Learning Resources

Resources Worth Building Into Regular Practice, Not Just Exam Preparation

PubMed, for direct literature searching — the single most reliable way to confirm whether a specific, current finding referenced anywhere, including in this book, remains the latest available evidence by the time you are reading it.

UpToDate or a comparable point-of-care clinical decision support tool, where institutionally available, for rapidly current, structured summaries of a specific clinical question during real patient care.

Your own institution's neonatal intensive care unit protocols and quality improvement committee materials — genuinely current, locally validated practice frequently reflects considerations a general textbook cannot fully capture.

National and regional neonatal networks, where you have access to one — this book's own Volume 4 has discussed at length why coordinated, networked benchmarking represents such an important, current quality improvement platform; the same networks are frequently a genuinely valuable, ongoing professional development resource.

Closing Note

Treat this list as a map, not a checklist to complete before sitting your examination. This book's own five volumes were built to be a complete, sufficient foundation on their own; the resources above are for the specific, individual questions this book leaves you wanting to chase further — during preparation, and for the entire career that follows it.

Reference Ranges Appendix

A Quick-Reference Companion to All Three Volumes

Vital Signs, Laboratory Values, Growth Parameters, Clinical Formulas, and Medication Reference

This appendix is built for a different purpose than the rest of this book. Every preceding chapter and mock examination was built to teach and to test. This appendix is built to be looked things up in — quickly, at the bedside, or while working back through a question you missed. It is deliberately terse: tables and numbers, with only as much surrounding text as a number needs to be used safely.

How Reference Ranges Actually Work

Every range in this appendix is a starting point for clinical judgement, not a substitute for it. Neonatal reference ranges vary by gestational age, postnatal age, and specific assay or laboratory, sometimes considerably. Where a range is genuinely gestational-age-dependent, this appendix says so explicitly and gives age-banded figures rather than a single, flattened number.

Always confirm a specific, individual result against your own institution's own local reference range and current assay methodology before treating it as abnormal. This appendix reflects widely used, general ranges compiled from standard neonatal reference sources; it does not replace institutional or manufacturer-specific values.

A Note on Figures

Every figure in this book is original artwork, drawn specifically for it. No stock images, no licensed photographs and no third-party illustrations are used anywhere in the text.

1. Vital Signs by Age

Heart rate, respiratory rate, and blood pressure all shift meaningfully across gestational and postnatal age. Use the band that most closely matches the individual infant.

1.1 Heart Rate (beats per minute, awake)

Population	Low	Typical range	High
Extremely preterm (<28 weeks)	100	120–180	200
Very preterm (28–31 weeks)	100	120–170	190
Moderate-late preterm (32–36 weeks)	100	110–160	180
Term, day 1–2	90	110–160	170
Term, week 1–4	100	110–150	170

1.2 Respiratory Rate (breaths per minute)

Population	Low	Typical range	High
Preterm, all gestations	30	40–60	70
Term, day 1–2	30	40–60	65
Term, week 1–4	25	30–55	60

A sustained rate above 60 at rest is tachypnoea in any neonate and warrants evaluation, regardless of gestational age.

1.3 Blood Pressure (mean arterial pressure, mmHg)

A widely used, general rule of thumb: mean arterial pressure in mmHg should approximate gestational age in weeks during the first days of life. This is a starting heuristic, not a validated formula — always interpret alongside perfusion, urine output, and lactate.

Gestational age	Systolic (mmHg)	Diastolic (mmHg)	Mean (mmHg)
24–26 weeks, day 1	35–54	20–33	24–36
27–29 weeks, day 1	38–56	23–36	28–38
30–32 weeks, day 1	41–60	25–38	30–41
33–36 weeks, day 1	46–64	28–40	34–44
Term, day 1	55–75	35–45	45–55
Term, day 4+	65–85	40–55	50–62

1.4 Temperature and Oxygen Saturation

Parameter	Target range	Notes
Axillary temperature	36.5–37.5°C	Below 36.5°C is hypothermia; below 36.0°C is significant hypothermia requiring active rewarming.
Preductal SpO_2, first 10 minutes of life	Rising from ~60% at 1 min to ~90–95% by 10 min	Follow the NRP target-saturation curve during transition, not a single fixed number.
SpO_2, stable preterm infant on supplemental oxygen	90–95%	Current evidence supports this range over higher targets; individualise per unit protocol.
SpO_2, stable term infant, room air	95–100%	Persistent values below 90% in room air warrant evaluation.

2. Haematology Reference Ranges

Haemoglobin, haematocrit, and white cell counts are all strongly age-dependent in the neonate, with a physiologic rise at birth followed by a nadir over subsequent weeks.

Parameter	Cord blood / Day 1	Day 3-7	Week 2-4 (term)	Notes
Haemoglobin (g/dL)	14–22	13–20	10–17	Physiologic nadir occurs around 8–12 weeks in term infants, earlier and lower in preterm infants.
Haematocrit (%)	42–65	40–62	31–55	Polycythaemia: haematocrit >65%. Significant anaemia: <35% central by day 1.
Reticulocyte count (%)	3–7	1–3	1–3	Elevated at birth reflecting active in utero erythropoiesis; falls sharply thereafter.
White cell count ($\times 10^9$/L)	9–30	5–21	5–19.5	Highly variable in the first 24 hours; trend matters more than a single value.
Absolute neutrophil count ($\times 10^9$/L)	1.8–5.4 (term, at birth)	1.0–9.0	1.5–8.5	Both neutropenia and neutrophilia occur physiologically; use a chart referenced to postnatal hours, not a flat cutoff.
Platelet count ($\times 10^9$/L)	150–450	150–450	150–450	Relatively stable across gestational age, unlike other cell lines. <100 warrants evaluation; <50 is severe.

2.1 Coagulation Parameters

Parameter	Term infant	Preterm infant	Notes
Prothrombin time (seconds)	13–20	14–22	Physiologically prolonged relative to older children given developmental immaturity of vitamin K-dependent factors.
Activated partial thromboplastin time (seconds)	30–55	35–70	Considerably wider, more prolonged normal range than in older children; interpret with this in mind before assuming coagulopathy.
Fibrinogen (g/L)	1.5–4.0	1.5–4.0	Broadly similar across gestational age.
Platelet count ($\times 10^9$/L)	150–450	150–450	See haematology table above.

3. Serum Chemistry Reference Ranges

Parameter	Reference range	Notes
Sodium (mmol/L)	133–146	Preterm infants may run several points lower in the first days given genuinely immature renal tubular handling.
Potassium (mmol/L)	3.7–6.0 (venous)	Higher upper limit than older children; true hyperkalaemia (>7.0) still requires action, but mild elevation is common and often non-pathologic in the first 24–48 hours, especially in preterm infants.
Chloride (mmol/L)	96–111	
Bicarbonate (mmol/L)	18–24 (term); 16–22 (preterm)	Genuinely lower normal range in preterm infants reflects immature renal bicarbonate reabsorption — see Volume 1's acid-base chapter.
Blood urea nitrogen (mg/dL)	3–12	Lower than older children/adults; rises with genuine dehydration, renal impairment, or excess protein load.
Creatinine (mg/dL), day 1	0.6–1.2 (reflects maternal value)	Falls over the first 1–2 weeks as maternal creatinine clears and this infant's own renal function matures.
Creatinine (mg/dL), week 2–4	0.2–0.4 (term); 0.3–0.6 (preterm)	A value that fails to fall, or that rises, after the first week is genuinely concerning regardless of the absolute number.
Glucose (mg/dL)	45–96	Significant neonatal hypoglycaemia is generally defined as <45 mg/dL in the first 24 hours, though operational thresholds vary by protocol and clinical context.

Parameter	Reference range	Notes
Calcium, total (mg/dL)	7.5–10.5 (term); 6.5–9.5 (preterm)	Physiologic nadir around 24–48 hours of life.
Calcium, ionised (mg/dL)	4.0–5.5	The more clinically reliable measure, especially in a sick or preterm infant.
Magnesium (mg/dL)	1.5–2.8	
Phosphorus (mg/dL)	4.5–9.0 (term); 5.5–9.5 (preterm)	Higher requirement in the preterm infant — see Volume 4's metabolic bone disease content.
Alkaline phosphatase (U/L)	110–320 (term); up to 900 in preterm infants with active bone mineralisation	A markedly elevated value with radiographic osteopenia suggests metabolic bone disease of prematurity.
Total bilirubin (mg/dL)	See age-specific phototherapy nomograms	Never interpreted as a flat cutoff — always plot against postnatal age in hours and specific risk factors.
Direct (conjugated) bilirubin (mg/dL)	<1.0, or <20% of total	A direct fraction exceeding 20% of total, or exceeding 1.0 mg/dL outright, warrants active evaluation for a cholestatic process.
Albumin (g/dL)	2.5–4.0	Lower than older children; genuinely lower in preterm infants.
Ammonia (µmol/L)	<110 (term); <150 (preterm, first days)	A markedly elevated value in an encephalopathic infant should prompt urgent evaluation for an inborn error of metabolism — see the critical sample principle in Volume 1.

4. Blood Gas Reference Ranges

Parameter	Arterial	Venous / capillary	Notes
pH	7.30–7.40	7.30–7.38	Lower limit of acceptable in a stable infant is generally 7.25; below 7.20 is significant acidaemia.
PCO_2 (mmHg)	35–45	40–50	See Volume 1's acid-base chapter and Volume 4's permissive hypercapnia content for target ranges in the ventilated preterm infant, which run genuinely higher.
PO_2 (mmHg)	50–80 (arterial, on room air or minimal support)	30–40	Target ranges vary considerably with clinical context and supplemental oxygen; interpret alongside SpO_2 trend, not in isolation.
Bicarbonate (mmol/L)	18–24	18–24	Genuinely lower in preterm infants — see the chemistry table above.
Base excess (mmol/L)	−4 to +4	−4 to +4	A base deficit beyond −8 to −10 suggests significant, active metabolic acidosis requiring evaluation for an underlying cause.
Lactate (mmol/L)	0.5–2.2	0.5–2.2	A rising, rather than a single, static value is the more clinically important signal; trend it during any evolving,

Parameter	Arterial	Venous / capillary	Notes
			concerning presentation.

5. Cerebrospinal Fluid Reference Ranges

Neonatal CSF reference ranges are genuinely, considerably wider than in older children, and preterm infants run higher normal values across nearly every parameter — a frequent source of diagnostic error if adult or paediatric ranges are applied by habit.

Parameter	Term infant	Preterm infant	Notes
White cell count (cells/µL)	0–22	0–25	Values up to 20–30 can be normal in an otherwise well-appearing neonate — correlate with the full, connected clinical picture, not this number alone.
Protein (mg/dL)	20–170	65–150 (up to 300 in very preterm infants)	Considerably higher than in older children at every gestational age; a genuinely elevated value alone does not confirm meningitis.
Glucose (mg/dL)	34–69 (generally 60–80% of serum glucose)	24–63	Interpret relative to a simultaneous serum glucose, not as an isolated, absolute number.
Red blood cells (cells/µL)	0- several hundred (traumatic tap common)	0- several hundred	A traumatic tap can meaningfully confound white cell count and protein interpretation — apply a correction factor or repeat the tap when genuinely in doubt.

6. Growth Parameters

Use a validated, gestational-age-specific growth chart (such as Fenton or INTERGROWTH-21st) for actual clinical plotting. The figures below are approximate, 50th-percentile reference points only, intended for quick orientation rather than formal growth assessment.

Gestational age at birth	Approximate weight (50th %ile)	Approximate length	Approximate head circumference
24 weeks	650–700 g	31–32 cm	21–22 cm
28 weeks	1100–1200 g	36–37 cm	25–26 cm
32 weeks	1700–1800 g	41–42 cm	29–30 cm
36 weeks	2600–2700 g	47–48 cm	32–33 cm
40 weeks (term)	3300–3400 g	50–51 cm	34–35 cm

Expected postnatal weight gain, once growth has stabilised: approximately 15–20 g/kg/day for a preterm infant on full enteral feeds; approximately 20–30 g/day (absolute) for a term infant in the first months. Weight loss of up to 7–10% in the first week is generally physiologic in a term infant regaining birthweight by 10–14 days; a preterm infant may lose up to 10–15% before beginning to regain.

7. Clinical Formulas and Calculations

Every formula below has appeared, applied to a specific clinical scenario, somewhere across this book's five volumes. This section collects them together as a single, quick-reference point.

Calculation	Formula	Clinical use
Corrected (adjusted) age	Chronological age – (40 weeks – gestational age at birth)	Used for growth and developmental assessment through approximately 2-3 years of age in an infant born preterm.
Oxygenation index	(Mean airway pressure × FiO_2 × 100) ÷ PaO_2	A rising value reflects worsening respiratory failure severity; used in ECMO candidacy assessment — see Volume 4.
Alveolar-arterial oxygen gradient	A–a gradient = [(Patm – PH_2O) × FiO_2 – ($PaCO_2$ ÷ 0.8)] – PaO_2	A widened gradient suggests a parenchymal or diffusion problem rather than pure hypoventilation.
Anion gap	$Na^+ - (Cl^- + HCO_3^-)$	Normal range approximately 8–16 mmol/L. An elevated gap suggests an unmeasured acid — lactate, an inborn error of metabolism, or renal failure — see Volume 1's acid-base chapter.
Fractional excretion of sodium (FENa)	(Urine Na × Plasma Cr) ÷ (Plasma Na × Urine Cr) × 100	Interpretation is genuinely age- and gestation-dependent in the neonate, unlike in older children; a value considered pathologic in an older child may be physiologic in a very preterm infant.
Number needed to treat	1 ÷ Absolute risk reduction	See Volume 4's biostatistics chapter — a lower number reflects a more powerful treatment effect.

Calculation	Formula	Clinical use
Absolute risk reduction	Control group event rate − Intervention group event rate	The genuine, actual difference in risk, distinct from relative risk reduction — see Volume 4.
Mean arterial pressure (from cuff)	Diastolic + [(Systolic − Diastolic) ÷ 3]	A rough estimate; direct arterial line measurement is more reliable when available.
Estimated maintenance fluid (day-of-life-based)	Day 1: ~60–80 mL/kg/day; increasing by ~15–20 mL/kg/day through the first week to ~120–150 mL/kg/day	Requires active, individual adjustment for gestational age, thermal environment, phototherapy, and clinical status.
Weight-based medication dosing (general)	Dose (mg) = Weight (kg) × Dose per kg	Always cross-check against a specific, current dosing reference — see Section 8 for selected examples discussed throughout this book.

8. Selected Medication Quick-Reference

This is a starting-point reference only, for the specific medications discussed at length across this book's five volumes. It is not a complete formulary and does not replace a current, institution-specific dosing reference or pharmacy consultation.

Medication	Typical indication	General dosing note	Key connected consideration
Caffeine citrate	Apnoea of prematurity	Loading ~20–25 mg/kg; maintenance ~5–10 mg/kg/day	Uniform weight-based dosing does not account for gestational-age-specific metabolism or renal function; genuinely current research links early exposure to AKI risk — see Volume 1.
Indomethacin	Haemodynamically significant PDA	~0.1–0.3 mg/kg/dose per protocol, typically 3 doses	Genuine renal risk, particularly with prolonged or repeated courses; associated with spontaneous intestinal perforation when combined with early corticosteroids — see Volumes 1 and 3.
Surfactant (poractant alfa or similar)	Surfactant-deficient respiratory distress syndrome	~100–200 mg/kg/dose via ETT or LISA technique	Can rapidly lower pulmonary vascular resistance, unmasking a previously silent PDA — see Volume 2.

Medication	Typical indication	General dosing note	Key connected consideration
Morphine (continuous infusion)	Procedural or postoperative analgesia	~5–20 µg/kg/hour, individually titrated	Infusions of approximately 5 days or longer carry genuine, significant withdrawal risk on discontinuation, requiring gradual weaning — see Volumes 1 and 3.
Midazolam	Sedation, often paired with an opioid	Continuous infusion generally preferred over bolus	Genuinely delayed neonatal elimination; particular caution with bolus dosing or opioid combination given associated hypotension risk — see Volume 1.
Prostaglandin E1	Maintaining ductal patency in duct-dependent cardiac lesions	Starting ~0.01–0.05 µg/kg/minute, continuous infusion	Apnoea is a recognised side effect; secure the airway plan before or promptly after initiation — see Volume 2.
Ampicillin + gentamicin (or similar)	Empiric early-onset sepsis coverage	Per current institutional and gestational-age-adjusted protocol	Dosing intervals are genuinely gestational- and postnatal-age-dependent given evolving renal clearance — see Volume 2.
Sodium bicarbonate	Selected, specific metabolic acidosis (not first-line)	Individualised; correct the underlying cause first	Correcting the underlying cause, not bicarbonate alone, is the

Medication	Typical indication	General dosing note	Key connected consideration
			correct, primary approach — see Volume 1's acid-base chapter.
Vitamin K (phytonadione)	Prevention of vitamin K deficiency bleeding	1 mg IM, single dose at birth (term); weight-adjusted in preterm infants	Universal, standard practice; oral alternatives carry a genuinely less reliable, established evidence base.
Acyclovir (intravenous)	Suspected or confirmed neonatal HSV infection	~20 mg/kg/dose IV, dosing interval per gestational and postnatal age	Prompt initiation is time-sensitive given genuine risk of rapid progression — see Volume 2.

9. Common Abbreviations Used Throughout This Book

Abbreviation	Meaning
AGA	Appropriate for gestational age
BPD	Bronchopulmonary dysplasia
CDH	Congenital diaphragmatic hernia
CPAP	Continuous positive airway pressure
CRIB / CRIB-II	Clinical Risk Index for Babies
ECMO	Extracorporeal membrane oxygenation
FENa	Fractional excretion of sodium
GBS	Group B Streptococcus
HIE	Hypoxic-ischaemic encephalopathy
IUGR	Intrauterine growth restriction
IVH	Intraventricular haemorrhage
LGA	Large for gestational age
NEC	Necrotising enterocolitis
NICU	Neonatal intensive care unit
NRP	Neonatal Resuscitation Program
OI	Oxygenation index
PDA	Patent ductus arteriosus
PPHN	Persistent pulmonary hypertension of the newborn
PVL	Periventricular leukomalacia
RDS	Respiratory distress syndrome
ROP	Retinopathy of prematurity

Abbreviation	Meaning
SGA	Small for gestational age
TTN	Transient tachypnoea of the newborn
VACTERL	Vertebral, Anal, Cardiac, Tracheo-oEsophageal, Renal, Limb association
VLBW / ELBW	Very low birthweight (<1500 g) / Extremely low birthweight (<1000 g)

Closing Note

This appendix closes the entire, five-volume Neonatal-Perinatal Board Review Question Bank. It was built as a companion to be returned to — during study, during a mock examination, and afterward, at the bedside. The numbers in it will need periodic updating as institutional protocols and assays evolve; the reasoning method taught throughout the preceding chapters will not.

Dr. Ahmed Badawy, MRCPCH.UK | EBP | EPIC — Talented LLC, Wyoming, USA — ORCID 0009-0007-7662-840X

Afterword

This closes the entire, five-volume Neonatal-Perinatal Board Review Question Bank. Across more than two thousand questions, seventeen clinical chapters, three complete mock examinations, and the preparation guidance in this closing volume, one method has run throughout: mechanism first, honest about uncertainty, and connected — across every chapter and every volume. Carry that method into the examination, and into the practice that follows it.

Author Contact and Publication Information

Correspondence: Dr. Ahmed Badawy. Email: a.m.b.hassane@gmail.com

Researcher identifiers: ORCID 0009-0007-7662-840X.

Series title: Neonatal-Perinatal Board Review Question Bank, Volume 5 of 5. First Edition, 2026.

Subject classification: Medical / Pediatrics / Neonatology; Medical / Test Preparation & Review; Medical / Critical Care.

Intended readership: Neonatal-perinatal medicine fellows and candidates preparing for subspecialty certifying examinations; general pediatric residents rotating through neonatal intensive care; advanced neonatal nurse practitioners.

Publisher: Talented LLC, Sheridan, Wyoming, USA.

For permissions, feedback, or collaboration enquiries, please write to the correspondence address above.

www.ingramcontent.com/pod-product-compliance
Lightning Source LLC
La Vergne TN
LVHW081736071126
851857LV00042B/1887
9798952203099